WORKBOOK FOR

PHARMACOLOGY FOR NURSES

A Pathophysiologic Approac'

FIRST EDITION

MICHAEL PATRICK ADAMS, PhD, RT(R)

Associate Dean of Health, Mathematics, and Science
Pasco-Hernando Community College

LELAND NORMAN HOLLAND, JR., PhD

Associate Academic Dean
Southeastern University

PEARSON
Prentice
Hall

Upper Saddle River, New Jersey

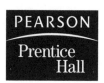

Notice: Care has been taken to confirm the accuracy of information presented in this textbook. The authors, editors, and publisher, however, cannot accept responsibility for errors or omissions or for consequences from application of the information in this textbook and make no warranty, expressed or implied, with respect to its contents.

The authors and publisher have exerted every effort to ensure that drug selections and dosages set forth in this textbook are in accord with current recommendations and practices at the time of publication. However, in view of ongoing research, changes in government regulations, and the constant flow of information relating to drug therapy and drug reactions, the reader is urged to check the package inserts of all drugs for any change in indications of dosage and for added warnings and precautions. This is particularly important when the recommended agent is a new and/or infrequently employed drug.

Publisher: Julie Levin Alexander
Assistant to the Publisher: Regina Bruno
Editor-in-Chief: Maura Connor
Executive Editor: Barbara Krawiec
Assistant Editor: Sladjana Repic
Developmental Editor: Elena M. Mauceri
Editorial Assistant: Jennifer Dwyer
Director of Production and Manufacturing: Bruce Johnson
Managing Production Editor: Patrick Walsh
Production Liaison: Mary C. Treacy
Production Editor: Amy Hackett, Carlisle Communications
Manufacturing Manager: Ilene Sanford
Manufacturing Buyer: Pat Brown
Design Director: Cheryl Asherman
Senior Design Coordinator: Maria Guglielmo Walsh
Senior Marketing Manager: Nicole Benson
Marketing Assistant: Janet Ryerson
Channel Marketing Manager: Rachele Triano
Composition: Carlisle Publisher Services
Cover Printer: Lehigh Press
Printer/Binder: Courier/Westford

Pearson Education LTD.
Pearson Education Singapore, Pte, Ltd
Pearson Education, Canada, Ltd
Pearson Education—Japan

Pearson Education Australia PTY, Limited
Pearson Education North Asia Ltd
Pearson Educación de Mexico, S.A. de C.V.
Pearson Education Malaysia, Pte. Ltd

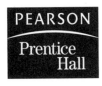

10 9 8 7 6 5 4 3
ISBN 0-13-028289-8

CONTRIBUTORS

Ellise D. Adams, CNM, MSN, CD(DONA), ICCE
Nursing Faculty
Calhoun Community College
Decatur, Alabama

Carol Ann Alexander, MSN, RN
Associate Professor
Palm Beach Community College
Lake Worth, Florida

Darcus Margarette Kottwitz, MSN, RN
Nursing Instructor
Fort Scott Community College
Fort Scott, Kansas

Janelle Hernden Sorrell, RN, BS
Instructor, Practical Nursing Program
Northwest-Shoals Community College
Muscle Shoals, Alabama

Jonna Swithers White, MSN, RN
Assistant Professor of Nursing
Tennessee State University, School of Nursing
Nashville, Tennessee

Patricia Moran Woodbery, BSN, MSN, ARNP-CS
Professor of Nursing
Valencia Community College
Orlando, Florida

REVIEWERS

Pattie Clark, RN, MSN
Associate Professor of Nursing
Abraham Baldwin College
Tifton, Georgia

Bill Farnsworth, RN, MSN, ABD
Clinical Instructor of Nursing
University of Texas at El Paso School of Nursing
El Paso, Texas

Catherine B. Kaesberg, MS, RN
Associate Instructorial Professor
Mennonite College at Illinois State University
Normal, Illinois

Barbara McNeill, RN, MSN
Associate Professor
College of Lake County
Grayslake, Illinois

CONTENTS

PREFACE

Pharmacology is one of the most challenging subjects for those embarking on careers in nursing. It is an interdisciplinary subject borrowing concepts from a wide variety of natural and applied sciences. The purpose of this workbook is to help you—the student—identify the essential content and master the critical concepts found in *Pharmacology for Nurses: A Pathophysiologic Approach, First Edition,* by Adams et al.

At the beginning of each chapter in this workbook, you will find a MediaLink box. Just as in the main textbook, this box identifies for you the specific media resources and activities available for that chapter on the CD-ROM, found in the main textbook and the Companion Website. You will find references to animations from the CD-ROM, and case studies and care plans from the Companion Website to help you visualize and comprehend difficult concepts. Chapter by chapter, this MediaLink box hones your critical-thinking skills and enables you to apply concepts from the textbook into practice.

In addition, each chapter includes a variety of questions and activities to help you comprehend difficult concepts and reinforce basic knowledge gained from textbook reading assignments. Highlights of this workbook that will enhance your learning experience include:

- The workbook chapters correlate directly to *Pharmacology for Nurses: A Pathophysiologic Approach, First Edition,* which allows you to easily locate information related to each question.
- Thorough assessment of essential information in the textbook is provided through the generous use of multiple choice, fill-in, and matching style questions in every chapter.
- Making Connections questions encourage you to recall concepts from previous chapters and apply them to the current chapter, thus promoting retention of information and continuity of learning.
- Dosage calculation problems provide additional practice to assist you in mastering this challenging topic.
- Clinical case studies provide in-depth scenarios to sharpen critical-thinking skills.
- Answers are included in the appendix to provide immediate reinforcement and to permit you to check the accuracy of your work.

It is our hope that this workbook contributes to the success of you beginning the study of an exciting and challenging subject.

CHAPTER 1

INTRODUCTION TO PHARMACOLOGY: DRUG REGULATION AND APPROVAL

OBJECTIVES

To view the objectives, please refer to the textbook, student CD-ROM, and the Companion Website at *www.prenhall.com/adams*.

FILL IN THE BLANK

From the textbook, find the correct word(s) to complete the statement(s).

1. The oldest form of healthcare is _____ therapy.

2. _____ is the father of American pharmacology.

3. In the early days of pharmacology, _____ had to isolate _____ from scarce natural products to create drugs used to treat patients.

4. In the 20th century, chemists and pharmacologists learned to _____ their own drugs in the laboratory.

5. The central purpose of pharmacology focuses on _____ the quality of life.

6. Pharmacology is defined as the _____ of _____ .

7. Therapeutics is the branch of medicine concerned with the _____ of disease.

8. Pharmacotherapeutics is the application of drugs for the purpose of disease _____

   and _____ .

9. A drug is a chemical agent capable of producing _____ or _____ responses.

10. _____ drugs do not require a physician's order.

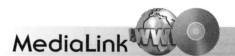

MediaLink

www.prenhall.com/adams

CD-ROM
Audio Glossary
NCLEX Review
Companion Website
NCLEX Review
Case Study
Expanded Key Concepts
Challenge Your Knowledge

MATCHING

For questions 11 through 14, match the concept in column I with the agent in column II.

Column I		Column II
11. _____	Biologics	a. Morphine
12. _____	Alternative therapies	b. Hormones
13. _____	Active agent	c. Herbs
14. _____	Nontherapeutic	d. Sunscreen

For questions 15 through 18, match the concept in column I with the definition in column II.

Column I		Column II
15. _____	Formulary	a. Standards for drugs
16. _____	Pharmacopeia	b. List of drugs
17. _____	USP label	c. Exact amount of ingredient
18. _____	Biologics Control Act	d. Drug regulation

MULTIPLE CHOICE

19. The Pure Food and Drug Act of 1906 gave the government power to do what action?

    a. Sell OTC products

    b. Synthesize morphine

    c. Control drug labeling

    d. Open pharmacy companies

20. The Food, Drug and Cosmetic Act of 1938 prevented which of the following actions?

    a. Use of herbal products

    b. Synthesis of narcotic substances

    c. Distribution of dietary supplements

    d. Sale of drugs that had not been thoroughly tested

21. The FDA is not responsible for overseeing the administration of which of the following products?

    a. Dietary supplements

    b. Herbal products

    c. OTC drugs

    d. Pesticides

22. Which of the following phases of drug approval produces inconclusive results?

    a. Clinical phase trials

    b. New drug application

    c. Preclinical investigation

    d. Postmarketing surveillance

23. In the drug approval process, what is the purpose of the postmarketing surveillance stage?

    a. Completion of laboratory tests on human cells

    b. Small clinical trials on volunteers

    c. Animal and human drug trials

    d. Survey for harmful effects in a large human population

24. What is the purpose of the Prescription Drug User Fee Act?

    a. To regulate use of dietary supplements

    b. To provide yearly user fees to the FDA

    c. To charge a lower fee to those who are chronically ill

    d. To allow elders to use drugs with greater freedom

25. Which of the following statements best describes an advantage of prescription drugs over OTC drugs?

    a. OTC drugs do not require a physician's order.

    b. Prescription drugs ensure that harmful reactions, ineffective treatment, or a progressive disease state will not occur.

    c. Only patients authorized to receive prescription drugs will take these medications.

    d. The nurse can maximize therapy by ordering the amount and frequency to be dispensed.

26. The Canadian Food and Drug Act regulates which of the following substances?

    a. Food

    b. Drugs

    c. Cosmetics

    d. All of the above

27. Which of the following statements is true about the drug approval process in Canada?

    a. Cosmetics do not need to be regulated.

    b. Homeopathic remedies need no formal regulation.

    c. Regulation is unnecessary if a drug has a drug identification number.

    d. The Canadian government needs to monitor natural dietary supplements and herbs.

28. Which of the following statements best describes the work of Health Canada?

    a. It is a federal department working to ensure proper management of health and safety issues.

    b. It represents pharmaceutical companies to speed the drug review process.

    c. It tests the potential for harmful drug effects on the general population.

    d. It enforces a drug user fee on pharmaceutical companies.

CASE STUDY APPLICATIONS

29. Mr. A has a problem with mild constipation. This symptom has just occurred and does not seem to be related to a major illness. He has considered trying OTC drugs such as Ex-Lax or Metamucil. He is also considering some natural alternative therapies.

   a. Using your knowledge of pharmacology, what teaching plan would you implement for Mr. A?

   b. What nursing history is important when answering Mr. A's questions.

30. Ms. B reports to you that she is experiencing a drug reaction. She states that she may have taken a generic medication that does not meet the standard for all pharmaceutical products.

   a. As a nurse, what assessment data are essential in the initial phase of the nurse-patient relationship with Ms. B?

   b. What would you teach Ms. B about drug regulations and standards?

CHAPTER 2

DRUG CLASSES AND SCHEDULES

OBJECTIVES

To view the objectives, please refer to the textbook, student CD-ROM, and the Companion Website at *www.prenhall.com/adams*.

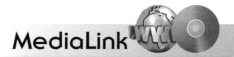

MediaLink

www.prenhall.com/adams

CD-ROM
Audio Glossary
NCLEX Review
Companion Website
NCLEX Review
Case Study

FILL IN THE BLANK

From the textbook, find the correct word(s) to complete the statement(s).

1. With _____ classifications, drugs are organized on the basis of their usefulness in treating a particular disorder.

2. Drugs organized by _____ classifications are categorized based on how they produce their effects in the body.

3. A _____ drug is the original, well-understood drug model from which other drugs in a therapeutic class have been developed.

4. The three types of drug names are _____ , _____ , and _____ names.

5. The description given to a drug by the International Union of Pure and Applied Chemistry (IUPAC) is its _____ name.

6. The _____ name for a drug is assigned by the manufacturer.

7. Drugs with more then one active ingredient are called _____ .

8. One of the main arguments against substituting generic drugs for brand name drugs is differences in _____ .

9. For the drug diphenhydramine (Benadryl), _____ is the generic name.

10. Brand name drugs are usually more _____ than their generic equivalent.

MATCHING

For questions 11 through 14, match the concept in column I with the concept in column II.

	Column I		Column II
11. _____	Pharmacologic classification	a.	Antihypertensive
12. _____	Therapeutic classification	b.	Calcium channel blocker
13. _____	Generic name	c.	Brand name
14. _____	Trade name	d.	Active ingredients

MULTIPLE CHOICE

15. What is the key to the therapeutic classification of a drug?

    a. Determine molecular changes that occur

    b. Clearly state what a drug does chemically

    c. Evaluate the body system affected by the drug

    d. Identify tissue changes that result after the medication is absorbed

16. A drug's trade name is assigned by what agency?

    a. FDA

    b. U.S. Adopted Name Council

    c. Developing pharmaceutical company

    d. International Union of Pure and Applied Chemistry

17. Which of the following statements best explains why a drug would be placed on the negative drug formulary list?

    a. Absorption of the drug affects drug action.

    b. Distribution of the drug to the target cells is prolonged.

    c. Bioavailability is different and affects drug uptake.

    d. Generic drug bioavailability is different from the brand name and affects patient outcomes.

18. Why is a drug classified as a scheduled drug?

    a. The drug can cause dependency.

    b. Alcohol is part of the drug composition.

    c. Generic and brand name drugs have different bioavailability.

    d. The generic drug company still has exclusive rights to production.

19. Which of the following substances requires classification as a scheduled drug?

    a. Vodka

    b. Morphine

    c. Benadryl

    d. Cigarettes

20. Which of the following schedule classifications has the highest potential for abuse?

    a. Schedule I

    b. Schedule II

    c. Schedule III

    d. Schedule IV

21. Which of the following schedule classifications has the sole purpose of use as a research agent?

    a. Schedule I

    b. Schedule II

    c. Schedule III

    d. Schedule IV

22. In the United States, what law restricts the use of controlled substances?

    a. FDA

    b. U.S. Pharmacopeia

    c. U.S. Adopted Name Council

    d. Controlled Substances Act

23. In Canada, which of the following drugs is not restricted?

    a. Barbiturates

    b. Amphetamines

    c. Antidepressants

    d. Anabolic steroids

24. You are working with a client from Canada. His prescription bottle has a "C" on the container. You know this labeling is indicative of what fact about the drug?

    a. The drug must be in a closed container.

    b. The container is filled with a narcotic drug.

    c. Controlled substances are contained in the prescription bottle.

    d. Combination drugs have been used to formulate this drug.

CASE STUDY APPLICATION

25. You are giving a hospitalized patient her morning medications. The patient asks you why you are giving the generic form acetaminophen instead of the trade product, Tylenol. The patient asks if there is a difference between trade and generic products.

    a. What is your best reply?

    b. The patient also asks if Tylenol is a controlled substance. What is your best reply?

CHAPTER 3

EMERGENCY PREPAREDNESS

OBJECTIVES

To view the objectives, please refer to the textbook, student CD-ROM, and the Companion Website at *www.prenhall.com/adams*.

FILL IN THE BLANK

From the textbook, find the correct word(s) to complete the statement(s).

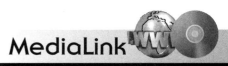

MediaLink

www.prenhall.com/adams

CD-ROM
Audio Glossary
NCLEX Review
Companion Website
NCLEX Review
Case Study

1. Traditional infectious diseases include possible epidemics caused

   by _____ , _____ , _____ , and _____ .

2. The program designed to supply essential medical equipment to a community in the event of a disaster is

   called _____ .

3. _____ are fully stocked sets of preassembled supplies that can be sent to a community in the United States within 12 hours after a bioterrorist attack.

4. Anthrax is normally seen in animals that have _____ .

5. Anthrax vaccine causes the body to make _____ which prevent the onset of disease.

6. Nerve agent antidote injector kits contain the anticholinergic drug _____ .

7. Potassium iodide is effective in preventing radiation-induced thyroid cancer even if taken _____ after radiation exposure.

MATCHING

For questions 8 through 14, match the information in column I with its disease in column II.

Column I	**Column II**
8. _____ Found in contaminated animal products such as wool, hair, bonemeal	a. Anthrax
9. _____ Oral vaccine available	b. Smallpox
10. _____ Caused by variola virus	c. Polio
11. _____ Genetic code is public information	
12. _____ Ciprofloxacin used for prophylaxis	
13. _____ Can be manufactured in a simple laboratory	
14. _____ Could cause mortality rate of up to 33% if released into unvaccinated population	

For questions 15 through 22, match the chemical agent in column II with the treatment in column I.

Column I	**Column II**
15. _____ Atropine	a. Nerve agents (sarin, soman, tabun)
16. _____ Give milk to drink	b. Lewisite
17. _____ Sodium thiosulfate 1% to induce emesis	c. Phosgene (gas)
18. _____ Fresh air and oxygen	d. Hydrogen cyanide
19. _____ Rinse nose and throat with 10% solution of sodium bicarbonate	e. Adamsite-DM
20. _____ Treat skin with borated talcum powder	
21. _____ Treat skin with 10% solution of sodium carbonate	
22. _____ Oxygen and amyl nitrate	

MULTIPLE CHOICE

23. Which of these is *not* an area of concern for possible use by bioterrorists?

    a. Infectious diseases such as anthrax and plague

    b. Incapacitating chemicals such as nerve gas and cyanide

    c. Common drugs such as morphine and strong antibiotics

    d. Nuclear and radiation exposures

24. When do the symptoms of anthrax exposure usually appear?

    a. 1 to 6 days after exposure

    b. 2 to 10 days after exposure

    c. 12 to 24 hours after exposure

    d. 1 week to 1 month after exposure

25. The public is discouraged from using antibiotics prophylactically unless there is a confirmed exposure to anthrax. All of the following are rationales for this policy except:

    a. Unnecessary use of antibiotics can be expensive

    b. Antibiotics can cause significant side effects

    c. Unnecessary use of antibiotics promotes the development of resistant bacteria

    d. Antibiotic use may inactivate the anthrax vaccine

26. Smallpox vaccine is contraindicated for all of the following persons except:

    a. A 25-year-old who is HIV positive

    b. An individual who has already been exposed to the disease

    c. A nursing mother

    d. An individual with eczema

27. Exposure to any of the nerve agents can cause all of the following symptoms except:

    a. Respiratory failure and convulsions

    b. Severe nausea and vomiting

    c. Increased sweating and salivation

    d. Incontinence of urine and stool

28. Radiation sickness is also known as which of the following?

    a. Acute radiation exposure

    b. Acute radiation syndrome

    c. Nuclear exposure syndrome

    d. Radioisotope syndrome

29. Which of the effects of radiation exposure may be prevented if potassium iodide is used within 3 to 4 hours of exposure to ionizing radiation?

    a. Leukemia

    b. Nausea, vomiting, diarrhea

    c. Thyroid cancer

    d. Bone marrow suppression

30. The 2001 JCAHO standards for emergency management include all of the following except:

    a. Response to immediate casualties

    b. How an agency's healthcare delivery will change during a crisis

    c. Disposition of fatalities

    d. Coordination of agency's efforts with community resources

31. Which of the following statements regarding the role of the nurse in emergency preparedness is *not* correct?

    a. The nurse must maintain a current knowledge of emergency management related to bioterrorist activities.

    b. The nurse must be aware of the early signs and symptoms of chemical and biological agents, and their immediate treatment.

c. The nurse should be involved in developing emergency plans.

d. The nurse should prepare for bioterrorist activities by receiving all available vaccines against biological agents.

32. *Bacillus anthracis* can be transmitted in all of the following ways except:

a. Bite by an insect that carries the disease

b. Exposure through an open wound

c. Contaminated food

d. Inhalation

CASE STUDY APPLICATIONS

33. During a routine visit to her doctor, Mrs. M confides to you that she is "terrified" of getting anthrax, even though no new cases have been reported in quite some time. She wants a supply of drugs to prevent an infection. You note that she becomes agitated while discussing terrorism, wringing her hands and looking distressed. Your nursing diagnosis is "Knowledge deficit related to bioterrorism/anthrax as evidenced by questions voiced and nonverbal anxiety behaviors."

    a. Your care plan includes interventions relating to patient education. What information would you give Mrs. M regarding prophylactic use of antibiotics for bioterrorism agents?

    b. What information would you give her about anthrax vaccine?

34. You are asked to assist in the writing of a protocol for the administration of smallpox vaccine to healthcare workers and law enforcement personnel in your area.

    a. What nursing assessments would be included prior to the administration of the vaccine?

    b. What information should be included in a pamphlet handed to each person who plans to be vaccinated?

35. Mr. R lives within 2 miles of a nuclear power plant. He comes to the doctor's office to request "the pills that make you immune to radiation sickness." Because you are aware that nurses play a key role in educating the public regarding bioterrorism, you have developed a standard care plan regarding nuclear disaster education for patients who live near the power plant.

    a. What patient teaching should you give to Mr. R regarding potassium iodide?

    b. In evaluating Mr. R's understanding of the information he has been given, you ask him to explain why potassium iodide is effective in preventing thyroid cancer after radiation exposure. What should be his answer?

CHAPTER 4

PRINCIPLES OF DRUG ADMINISTRATION

OBJECTIVES

To view the objectives, please refer to the textbook, student CD-ROM, and the Companion Website at *www.prenhall.com/adams*.

FILL IN THE BLANK

From the textbook, find the correct word(s) to complete the statement(s).

1. The_____ route means the nurse will administer the drug to the patient by mouth, under the tongue, or into the rectum.

2. When the nurse places a drug directly onto the skin or associated membranes, this is referred to as the _____ route.

3. The _____ phase of drug delivery involves four processes in the body: absorption, distribution, metabolism, and excretion.

4. _____ and _____ are two physical properties of a liquid drug that influence its movement throughout the body.

5. Drugs swallowed, chewed, or slowly dissolved in the mouth are referred to as _____ medications.

6. _____ administration involves placing drugs under the tongue.

7. _____ and _____ are examples of rectal administration methods.

8. The most common parenteral method of drug delivery is the _____ route.

9. Drugs are injected directly into the muscle in the _____ route.

10. An _____ injection is made directly into the spinal subarachnoid space; an _____ injection is made into the space overlying the dura mater.

www.prenhall.com/adams

CD-ROM
Audio Glossary
NCLEX Review
Companion Website
NCLEX Review
Case Study
Expanded Key Concepts
Challenge Your Knowledge

11. One popular method for delivering drugs across the skin at a slow steady rate is the _____ patch.

12. _____ drug delivery methods are useful in treating respiratory and reproductive ailments.

MATCHING

For questions 13 through 23, match the specific drug delivery method in column I with its general route in column II.

	Column I	**Column II**
13. _____	Rectal	a. Enteral
14. _____	Intravenous (IV)	b. Parenteral
15. _____	Intramuscular (IM)	c. Topical
16. _____	Oral (PO)	
17. _____	Transmucosal	
18. _____	Subcutaneous (SC or SQ)	
19. _____	Transdermal	
20. _____	Sublingual	
21. _____	Intrathecal (IT)	
22. _____	Intradermal	
23. _____	Subarachnoid	

For questions 24 through 32, match the traditional drug formulation in column I with its physical composition in column II.

	Column I	**Column II**
24. _____	Inhalants	a. Solids
25. _____	Suppositories	b. Liquids and liquid mixtures
26. _____	Lozenges	c. Gases
27. _____	Drops	
28. _____	Creams	
29. _____	Aerosols	
30. _____	Capsules	
31. _____	Ointments	
32. _____	Tablets	

MULTIPLE CHOICE

33. Which of the following statements about dissolution should the nurse consider correct?

    a. The shorter the dissolution time, the more delayed the onset of action.

    b. Water, taken in combination with solid drug formulations, is meant only to help dissolve the drugs.

    c. The process of dissolving solid drugs is dissolution.

    d. Dissolution time is only important for the drug administration phase of drug delivery.

34. After being administered, a medication must then be absorbed to produce an effect. After the medication is absorbed, which phase of drug delivery is occurring?

    a. Pharmaceutical phase

    b. Pharmacokinetic phase

    c. Pharmacodynamic phase

    d. None of the above

35. Of the following patients, which would be appropriate for rectal administration?

    a. Unconscious patient

    b. Patient experiencing nausea or vomiting

    c. Infant who cannot swallow pills

    d. All of the above

36. Which of the following drug delivery methods is *not* a parenteral method of drug delivery, and avoids the first-pass effect in the liver?

    a. Oral

    b. Intrathecal

    c. Intramuscular

    d. Sublingual

37. Which of the following is a major advantage of IV drug administration?

    a. The duration of drug action can be easily controlled.

    b. It is relatively free from the possibility of harmful effects.

    c. A precise concentration of drug can be administered into the bloodstream.

    d. The onset of drug action can be easily controlled.

38. What is a disadvantage of subcutaneous drug delivery?

    a. The final drug concentration within the bloodstream is unpredictable.

    b. Drugs cannot be confined to a precise location.

    c. For safety reasons, patients must be conscious when they receive a subcutaneous injection.

    d. Pain, swelling, or infection may occur if proper precautions are not taken.

39. If rapid onset of action is critical, which of the following routes would the nurse choose?

    a. Intravenous

    b. Intramuscular

    c. Sublingual

    d. Rectal

40. Which of the following drug administration methods would the nurse use for the tuberculin test with purified protein derivative (PPD)?

    a. Topical

    b. Intradermal

    c. Subcutaneous

    d. Intramuscular

41. Implants are generally administered by which drug delivery method?

    a. Intradermal

    b. Subcutaneous

    c. Intraperitoneal

    d. Intramuscular

42. Which of the following drug delivery methods might be used when fast delivery to the cerebral spinal fluid is necessary?

    a. Intraperitoneal

    b. Intrathecal

    c. Epidural

    d. Transmucosal

43. Which of the following is true about the physical properties of drugs?

    a. Substances that are able to dissolve in lipids (fats) are called hydrophilic.

    b. Hydrophobic drugs mix well in the bloodstream but move less efficiently across body membranes.

    c. Drugs with lipid properties mix well with components of cellular membranes.

    d. All of the above are correct.

44. Which of the following statements is true about IV infusions?

    a. Single drug doses are generally administered over a shorter period of time.

    b. A flow regulator is always used to regulate drug flow.

    c. Quick delivery of IV drugs is not possible with IV infusion.

    d. Drug doses are generally administered by way of a syringe and needle.

45. What is the deepest skin layer?

    a. Epidermis

    b. Dermis

    c. Hypodermis

    d. Muscular layer

46. Which of the following statements is true regarding topical drug applications?

    a. For a local effect, it is necessary to keep drugs from penetrating the skin barrier.

    b. Liquids and liquid mixtures are the most effective physical compositions for topical drug therapy.

    c. In some cases it is desirable for topical drugs to enter the systemic circulation.

    d. All of the above are correct.

47. What is the most common type of drug formulation for eye and ear medications?

    a. Salves

    b. Ointments

    c. Drops

    d. Sprays

CASE STUDY APPLICATIONS

48. In some cases, many different formulations are available, giving patients more than one option for drug therapy. Birth control is an example. Patients may take birth control pills, receive injections, or take medication via transdermal patches or vaginal inserts. Each method has advantages and disadvantages. Consider a situation in which your patient, a 34-year-old working mother, has an active lifestyle and needs a reliable and effective means of birth control.

    a. What assessment data should be gathered?

    b. Outline the patient teaching necessary to help this patient make the best choice.

49. An elderly man presents with a complaint of nausea and diarrhea. After a thorough assessment, the physician determines that medication might help relieve some of these symptoms and requests the nurse to administer the medication.

    a. In planning drug administration routes, what would you recommend for this patient and why?

    b. How will the nurse evaluate effectiveness of this route of administration?

CHAPTER 5

PHARMACOKINETICS

OBJECTIVES

To view the objectives, please refer to the textbook, student CD-ROM, and the Companion Website at *www.prenhall.com/adams*.

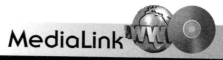

MediaLink

www.prenhall.com/adams

CD-ROM
Audio Glossary
NCLEX Review

Companion Website
NCLEX Review
Case Study
Expanded Key Concepts
Challenge Your Knowledge

FILL IN THE BLANK

From the textbook, find the correct word(s) to complete the statement(s).

1. The four main categories used to group processes relating to pharmacokinetics are _____ , _____ , _____ , and _____ .

2. The brain and placenta have barriers that prevent some medications from gaining access through normal circulation. These are the _____ and _____ barriers.

3. _____ is a process whereby most medications are deactivated when passing through the liver.

4. A mechanism called the _____ decreases the activity of most medications traveling through the liver.

5. _____ is a process involving the movement of a substance from its site of administration across body membranes to circulating fluids.

6. Four body tissues that have a high affinity for certain medications are _____ , _____ , _____ , and _____ .

7. Medications are removed from the body by the process of _____ .

8. _____ is the plasma level of a medication that will result in serious adverse effects for the patient.

9. The plasma drug concentration between the minimum effective concentration and the toxic concentration is called the _____ of the drug.

10. A _____ dose is a higher amount of drug given to "prime" the patient's bloodstream with a level of drug sufficient to quickly induce a therapeutic response.

MATCHING

For questions 11 through 14, match the factors affecting absorption in column I with the absorption/distribution rates shown in column II.

Column I	Column II
11. _____ Absence of food in the digestive tract	a. Faster absorption/distribution rate
12. _____ Binding of a drug to plasma proteins	b. Slower absorption/distribution rate
13. _____ Ability to mix with lipids	
14. _____ Larger drug particle	

MULTIPLE CHOICE

15. What is the process of moving a medication from its site of administration across one or more body membranes called?

    a. Absorption

    b. Distribution

    c. Metabolism

    d. Excretion

16. What process describes how drugs are transported in the body?

    a. Absorption

    b. Distribution

    c. Metabolism

    d. Excretion

17. What term describes how much of a drug is available to produce a biologic response?

    a. Volume of distribution

    b. Rate of elimination

    c. Bioavailability

    d. Half-life $(t_{1/2})$

18. The fact that the half-life $(t_{1/2})$ of drug A is longer than that of drug B might be explained by a higher:

    a. Metabolic rate for drug A

    b. Rate of elimination for drug B

    c. Potency for drug A

    d. Efficacy for drug B

19. Which of the following refers to the removal of larger drug metabolites from the bloodstream to the urine?

    a. Filtration

    b. Reabsorption

    c. Secretion

    d. Recirculation

20. Which of the following is a true statement regarding the half-life of a medication?

   a. The greater the half-life the longer the drug takes to be excreted.

   b. The longer the half-life of a drug the shorter the effect the drug will have on the body.

   c. Half-life and therapeutic range are terms that may be used interchangeably.

   d. When you know the loading dose you know the half-life of a drug.

21. When a drug is highly bound to protein complexes, what effect does that have for the patient?

   a. Drugs bound to protein are not available for distribution to body tissues.

   b. Highly bound drugs reach their target cells very quickly.

   c. These drugs cross the blood-brain barrier in minutes.

   d. Protein binding makes the drug more water soluble.

22. Which of the following routes of medication delivery *do not* bypass the first-pass effect?

   a. Rectal

   b. Sublingual

   c. Oral

   d. Parenteral

23. Which of the following body systems, if altered, could dramatically affect pharmacokinetics?

   a. Integumentary

   b. Musculoskeletal

   c. Sensory

   d. Renal

24. After drug therapy has been discontinued, what processes in the body contribute to the drug's presence in the body for several more weeks?

   a. Enterohepatic recirculation

   b. Integumentary elimination

   c. Respiratory elimination

   d. Renal excretion

CASE STUDY APPLICATIONS

25. Mr. P is anxious and has not been able to sleep well for several weeks. He is moderately obese and has a history of hypertension and diabetes. After examination, the healthcare practitioner agrees to provide this patient with a drug to treat anxiety.

   a. What assessment data support the fact that drug distribution could be a problem for this patient?

   b. How will the nurse evaluate the effectiveness of the drugs used to treat anxiety?

   c. What is the primary site for excretion of this patient's medications and therefore the system that must be consistently evaluated by the nurse?

26. Mr. A is 60 years old and has been abusing alcohol for years. He appears to have no major medical problems. He has been admitted to an outpatient setting for a diagnostic evaluation of his bowel by colonoscopy.

   a. What elements of his history would alert the nurse to possible problems with pharmacokinetics?

   b. What interventions might the nurse expect during the medication phase of this procedure?

   c. What system(s) should the nurse assess following the delivery of any medications for this patient?

CHAPTER 6

PHARMACODYNAMICS

OBJECTIVES

To view the objectives, please refer to the textbook, student CD-ROM, and the Companion Website at *www.prenhall.com/adams*.

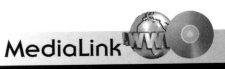

MediaLink

www.prenhall.com/adams

CD-ROM
Audio Glossary
Animation: Agonist
NCLEX Review

Companion Website
NCLEX Review
Case Study
Expanded Key Concepts
Challenge Your Knowledge

FILL IN THE BLANK

From the textbook, find the correct word(s) to complete the statement(s).

1. _____ deals with how medications affect body responses.

2. The classic theory about the cellular mechanism by which most medications produce a response is called the _____ theory.

3. _____ refers to a drug's strength at a particular concentration or dose, whereas _____ refers to the effectiveness of a drug in producing a more intense response as the concentration is increased.

4. A _____ curve is a graphical representation of the actual number of patients responding to a drug action at different doses.

5. The median effective dose (ED_{50}) is the dose required to produce a specific therapeutic response in _____ % of a group of patients.

6. The median lethal dose (LD_{50}) is the dose of drug that will be _____ in 50% of a group of animals.

7. A drug's _____ offers the nurse practical information on the safety of a drug.

8. A drug that is more potent will produce a therapeutic effect at a _____ dose, compared to another drug in the same class.

9. _____ is the magnitude of maximal response that can be produced from a particular drug.

10. _____ often compete with agonists for the receptor binding sites.

© 2005 by Pearson Education, Inc.

MATCHING

For questions 11 through 15, match the factors influencing drug effectiveness in column I with the area of pharmacokinetics or pharmacodynamics in column II.

Column I

11. _____ Concentration (dose) of an administered drug

12. _____ Presence of food in the digestive tract

13. _____ Frequency of drug dosing

14. _____ Age of the patient

15. _____ Kidney disease

Column II

a. pharmacokinetics

b. pharmacodynamics

MULTIPLE CHOICE

16. Which of the following best explains the pharmacodynamic phase of drug administration?

   a. The way the drug is absorbed, distributed, and eliminated from the body

   b. Drug action and the relationship between drug concentration and body responses

   c. Movement of substances from site of administration across body membranes

   d. First-pass effect which determines the frequency of dosing

17. You are giving a drug that is unfamiliar to you. You check the drug guide and determine that the average dose for the drug is 100 mg per day. Which of the following statements best explains what that means to you?

   a. The amount 100 mg will be the effective dosing for about 50% of the population.

   b. The amount 100 mg is the normal dose and it should be given twice per day.

   c. Few patients will respond to the 100 mg dose without side effects.

   d. Most patients will have a reaction if given more than 100 mg/day.

18. You are explaining to a patient the concept of drug potency. Which of the following statements best explains the concept?

   a. "If you are told to take a drug to control thyroid problems, the drug with the lowest milligram weight is the most potent."

   b. "A 100 mg dose is a more potent drug dosing then a 50 mg dose."

   c. "Dosing has nothing to do with potency. Site of injection is the most important part of dosing theory."

   d. "Your size and weight is what determines drug potency."

19. When drug molecules bind with cell receptors, what occurs?

   a. Pharmacologic effects of agonism or antagonism occur.

   b. Pharmacogenetics occurs quickly.

   c. The therapeutic index is increased.

   d. Potency of the drug is altered.

20. The pharmacist tells you that a drug has a high therapeutic index. Which of the following statements best reflects your understanding of that statement?

    a. Phase I of the dose response curve would be low.

    b. It is therapeutic to give this drug once per day.

    c. It would take a big error in dosing to create a lethal dose for this patient.

    d. I'd better be really careful, there are a lot of receptors that are sensitive to this drug.

21. Which pharmacologic principles will guide your practice as a nurse?

    a. Future medications may be customized to match the patient's genetic makeup.

    b. If you understand potency and efficacy, you can compare medications.

    c. As the therapeutic index increases, the safety of the drug increases.

    d. All of the above are true.

22. You are reviewing the terms *efficacy* and *potency* with a patient who is getting medications for cancer. What statement is most correct?

    a. "You need to be most interested in the number of milligrams the medication is going to provide. This is called potency."

    b. "The number of cancer cells killed is called efficacy. You are most interested in efficacy in the treatment of your disease."

    c. "Your cancer is going to require that the fewest numbers of receptors are affected. So, concentrate on potency."

    d. "Cancer is such a genetic issue. It is best to ask questions about dose and drug reactions, not efficacy."

23. The nurse hears in a report that a patient had an idiosyncratic reaction to a medication. Which of the following statements best explains what happened to the patient?

    a. No response, good or bad, was seen 24 hours after delivery of the medication.

    b. Drug-to-drug interaction occurred and less medication was needed.

    c. An unpredictable and unexplained drug reaction occurred.

    d. An antagonist reaction occurred at the receptor level.

24. Which statement best describes antagonists?

    a. They are sometimes referred to as facilitators of drug action.

    b. They can only produce an effect by interacting with receptors.

    c. They inhibit or block the action of agonist drugs.

    d. All of the above are correct.

25. You are giving two drugs to a patient with a heart problem. One drug works at the $beta_1$-adrenergic receptor and the other works at the $beta_2$-receptor. Which of the following statements bests explains how that can be possible?

    a. This is an example of potency and must be questioned.

    b. The graded dose response is the best explanation for this order.

    c. Lethal dose is determined on preclinical trials of beta-receptor drugs.

    d. The drugs are fine-tuned and can affect the different beta-receptor types in specific ways.

CASE STUDY APPLICATIONS

26. A patient with a history of severe migraines is taking an analgesic that is classified as an agonist/antagonist. The patient has not asked for the analgesic for 3 hours.

    a. What nursing assessment would you perform before giving this analgesic?

    b. What nursing diagnosis would you consider before giving this analgesic?

    c. What questions would you ask if the migraine headaches are not relieved within 15 minutes?

27. You are a nurse working with patients in an infectious disease clinic. Several of the patients are complaining that their wound infections are not healing quickly enough. You review their medical records.

    a. What information are you looking for related to pharmacotherapy?

    b. What outcomes would you expect to measure for the patient in a wound management clinic?

    c. What evaluation would support your recommendation for a medication change?

CHAPTER 7

DRUG ADMINISTRATION THROUGHOUT THE LIFESPAN

OBJECTIVES

To view the objectives, please refer to the textbook, student CD-ROM, and the Companion Website at *www.prenhall.com/adams*.

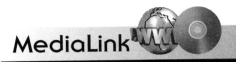

MediaLink

www.prenhall.com/adams

CD-ROM
Audio Glossary
NCLEX Review
Companion Website
NCLEX Review
Case Study
Expanded Key Concepts
Challenge Your Knowledge

FILL IN THE BLANK

From the textbook, find the correct word(s) to complete the statement(s).

1. A term that characterizes the progressive increase in physical size is _____ .

2. The functional evolution of the physical, psychomotor, and cognitive capabilities of a living being is referred to as _____ .

3. The whole-person theory is essential to _____ care.

4. The _____ period is subdivided into the _____ period (conception to 8 weeks) and the _____ period (8 to 40 weeks or birth).

5. During the _____ stage, nursing care and pharmacotherapy are directed toward safety of the infant, accurate dosing, and drug administration.

6. During the _____ stage, a child has a tremendous sense of curiosity and begins to try new things by placing them in the mouth.

7. The _____ -age child begins to refine gross and fine motor skills.

8. Thinking processes become progressively logical and more consistent in the _____ child.

9. During _____ , pharmacotherapy is for skin problems, headaches, menstrual symptoms, and sports-related injuries.

10. The taking of multiple drugs, or _____ , in older adults increases the risk for drug interactions and side effects.

MATCHING

For questions 11 through 15, match the pregnancy categories in column I with their descriptions in column II.

Column I

11. _____ Category A

12. _____ Category B

13. _____ Category C

14. _____ Category D

15. _____ Category X

Column II

a. Studies have *not* shown a risk to the mother or to the fetus.

b. Use of this drug *may* cause harm to the fetus, but it may provide benefit to the mother if a safer therapy is not available.

c. Animal studies *have* shown a risk to the fetus, but controlled studies have not been performed in women.

d. Studies *have* shown a significant risk to the mother and to the fetus.

e. Animal studies have *not* shown a risk to the fetus, or if they have, studies in women have not confirmed this risk.

MULTIPLE CHOICE

16. During the first trimester of pregnancy, what is (are) the primary consideration(s) from a medical, nursing, and pharmacologic viewpoint?

   a. Assessing and evaluating each patient on an individual basis, so that mistaken beliefs can be clarified

   b. Safety of the patient and delivery of a healthy baby

   c. Evaluating the knowledge base of the mother in regard to growth and development

   d. A focus on reducing the physical discomforts of the mother

17. The nurse determines that the fetus is at the greatest risk for developmental anomalies during which trimester?

   a. First

   b. Second

   c. Third

   d. Fourth

18. During which trimester do the skeleton and major organs develop?

   a. First

   b. Second

   c. Third

   d. Fourth

19. During a routine prenatal visit in her third trimester, a patient informs the nurse that she is smoking again because of a stressful situation at her job. The nurse counsels the patient on the increased risks to the fetus. Why are risks increased at this time?

    a. Blood flow to the placenta increases and placental vascular membranes become thinner.

    b. Drugs reaching the fetus have a reduced duration of action.

    c. The fetus receives reduced amounts of substances from the maternal bloodstream.

    d. Blood flow to the placenta decreases and placental vascular membranes become thicker.

20. The nurse is providing patient education in regard to breastfeeding. In relationship to drug and substance intake, what are the risks to the infant?

    a. Equal risks

    b. No risks

    c. Reduced risks

    d. Increased risks

21. What is the preferred site for administering an IM injection to an infant?

    a. Deltoid

    b. Dorsogluteal

    c. Gluteus maximus

    d. Vastus lateralis

22. When determining the correct method for calculating drug amount for infants, what must the nurse consider?

    a. Development of the immune system

    b. Development of the nervous system

    c. Age and size of the infant

    d. Infant's ability to swallow medications

23. When assessing risk factors, which age group must the nurse evaluate the patient's desire to explore and risks encountered?

    a. School-age

    b. Toddler

    c. Infant

    d. Preschool age

24. When assessing risk factors, which age group must the nurse evaluate the patient's development of gross and fine motor skills and the risks encountered?

    a. School-age

    b. Toddler

    c. Infant

    d. Preschool age

25. When assessing risk factors, which age group must the nurse evaluate the patient's concept of illness and potential to ingest any substance offered by a peer or older person and the risks encountered?

    a. School-age

    b. Toddler

    c. Infant

    d. Preschool age

26. During adolescence the nurse assumes a key role in the patient's education in relationship to which of the following?

    a. Use of vitamins

    b. Use of herbal remedies

    c. Use of prescription medications

    d. Use of tobacco and illicit drugs

27. During which period of adulthood would the nurse expect to offer counseling in relationship to substance abuse and sexually transmitted diseases?

    a. Middle adulthood

    b. Young adulthood

    c. Older adulthood

    d. None of the above

28. During which period of adulthood would the nurse expect to offer counseling in relationship to positive lifestyle modifications?

    a. Middle adulthood

    b. Young adulthood

    c. Older adulthood

    d. None of the above

29. During which period of adulthood would the nurse expect to offer counseling in relationship to increased potential for adverse reactions to medications related to physiologic and biochemical processes?

    a. Middle adulthood

    b. Young adulthood

    c. Older adulthood

    d. None of the above

30. The nurse knows that antidepressants and antianxiety agents are used more frequently by which age group?

    a. Over 65

    b. Over 50

    c. Over 40

    d. Over 30

MAKING CONNECTIONS

31. Which branch of medicine deals with the general treatment of suffering and disease?

    a. Pharmacotherapeutics

    b. Pathophysiology

    c. Therapeutics

    d. Physiology

32. What does the prototype approach to drug therapy consider?

    a. Most popular drug for a particular disorder

    b. Most commonly used drug in a particular class

    c. Representative drug for how other drugs in a particular class work

    d. Drug of choice for a particular disorder

33. What is the most common type of drug formulation for eye and ear medications?

    a. Salves

    b. Ointments

    c. Drops

    d. Sprays

34. For which sleep disorder drug do patients often fake or change prescriptions?

    a. Amphetamines

    b. Barbiturates

    c. Benzodiazepines

    d. Opioids

35. Which of the following drugs block the action of norepinephrine at alpha-and beta-receptors?

    a. Parasympathomimetics

    b. Parasympatholytics

    c. Sympathomimetics

    d. Sympatholytics

CASE STUDY APPLICATIONS

36. Ms. Y, age 19, presents to your clinic 20 weeks' pregnant. She has received no prenatal care, has a history of substance abuse, and admits to using tobacco, alcohol, and cocaine during her pregnancy. Based on your knowledge as a nurse, assess for the potential of developmental anomalies for the fetus. Also evaluate the potential for future complications if the substance abuse continues throughout the pregnancy.

    a. What are the potential anomalies in the fetus at the time of the visit?

    b. What are the potential complications to the pregnancy?

    c. State the rationale for the potential anomalies and complications.

37. Mrs. K is a 52-year-old mother of two grown children, six grandchildren, and aging parents with various health problems. She is married and her husband is disabled. Mrs. K also has a full-time job and two part-time jobs. When she presents to your clinic she is 50 pounds overweight and displays signs and symptoms of excessive stress. Evaluate the potential complications from this situation and emphasize changes in your patient education.

   a. What are middle-aged adults sometimes called?

   b. What options do these adults have to control their lifestyles?

   c. What health factors are often in place at this time in the life cycle?

38. Mr. Z, age 72, presents with a variety of health problems. He is presently taking 14 different medications prescribed by four different nurses. As the nurse in charge of patient education, assess the situation and determine the lifestyle changes that are necessary to ensure optional health for this patient.

   a. Taking multiple drugs concurrently is known by what term?

   b. How does this action affect drug interactions and potential for adverse reaction?

   c. What areas should the nurse assess carefully in this patient's health history?

CHAPTER 8

THE NURSING PROCESS IN PHARMACOLOGY

OBJECTIVES

To view the objectives, please refer to the textbook, student CD-ROM, and the Companion Website at *www.prenhall.com/adams*.

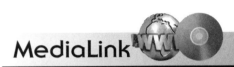

FILL IN THE BLANK

From the textbook, find the correct word(s) to complete the statement(s).

1. A _____ is taken during the initial meeting between a nurse and patient.

2. Problem-focused or "_____" history is taken to focus on the symptoms that prompted the patient to seek healthcare.

3. A _____ is also completed to gather objective data.

4. Nurses use their skills in _____ during the interview to collect data that is denied or downplayed.

5. The _____ is a systematic method of problem solving with clearly defined steps.

MATCHING

For questions 6 through 13, match the description in column I with the Nursing Process step in column II.

Column I	Column II
6. _____ First step in the Nursing Process	a. Evaluation
7. _____ Data that include what the patient says	b. Intervention
8. _____ Data gathered through diagnostic sources	c. Nursing diagnoses

© 2005 by Pearson Education, Inc.

9. _____ Provide the basis for planning patient care

10. _____ Objective measure of goals

11. _____ Links strategies to established outcomes

12. _____ Designed to ensure safe, effective care

13. _____ Assessment of goals and outcomes

d. Objective data

e. Subjective data

f. Assessment

g. Outcomes

h. Planning

MULTIPLE CHOICE

14. Mr. J has just returned from surgery. As the nurse, you are doing vital signs, checking his incision site, and determining if he is in pain. With these actions, what step of the Nursing Process are you using?

    a. Evaluation

    b. Planning

    c. Assessment

    d. Intervention

15. Mr. J has begun to complain of pain in his incision site. As the nurse, you are to administer morphine sulfate 2 mg IV. With these actions, what step of the Nursing Process are you using?

    a. Evaluation

    b. Planning

    c. Assessment

    d. Intervention

16. Mr. J has inquired about the physical therapy he will be receiving to regain his mobility after his knee replacement surgery. As the nurse, you will interact with physical therapy to coordinate his plan of care. With these actions, what step of the Nursing Process are you using?

    a. Evaluation

    b. Planning

    c. Assessment

    d. Intervention

17. Mr. J received the physical therapy and has regained his mobility after his knee replacement surgery. As the nurse, you interact with physical therapy to determine if he is ready to be discharged from the skilled unit. With these actions, what step of the Nursing Process are you using?

    a. Evaluation

    b. Planning

    c. Assessment

    d. Intervention

18. Ms. L is complaining of pain in her right hip. As the nurse, you have assessed the area and have found no swelling, redness, open areas, and there is no history of trauma to the hip. What type of information have you gathered?

    a. Objective data

    b. Subjective data

    c. Outcomes

    d. Goals

19. Ms. L is complaining of pain in her right hip. As the nurse, you have assessed the area and have found swelling, redness, open areas, and there is a history of trauma to the hip. What type of information have you gathered?

    a. Objective data

    b. Subjective data

    c. Outcomes

    d. Goals

20. Ms. L is complaining of pain in her right hip. As the nurse, you have assessed the area and have found swelling, redness, open areas, and there is a history of trauma to the hip. This information may be used to compare with assessment information gathered at a later date. What type of information have you gathered?

    a. Objective data

    b. Subjective data

    c. Outcomes

    d. Baseline data

21. Mrs. C is recovering from a fracture of the right hip. The interdisciplinary team has established a schedule of physical therapy for her. She will ambulate using a walker with the assist of one member of the team for 50 feet three times a day for 1 week, to be increased to 100 feet three times a day for 2 weeks, then to be changed to a quad cane and stand by assist for 2 weeks and then discharged to home. What type of information has been presented?

    a. Outcomes

    b. Goals

    c. Baseline data

    d. Objective data

22. Mrs. C is recovering from a fracture of the right hip. The interdisciplinary team has established a schedule of physical therapy for her. She is ambulating using a quad cane without assistance. It has been established she is ready to be discharged to her home. What type of information has been presented?

    a. Outcomes

    b. Goals

    c. Baseline data

    d. Subjective data

23. Using the information in question 21, select the priority nursing diagnosis for the patient.

    a. Pain R/T hip fracture AEB complaints of pain with ambulation

    b. Immobility R/T hip fracture AEB inability to stand or ambulate without assistance

    c. Knowledge deficit R/T hospitalization AEB first time in the hospital at 87 years of age

    d. Risk for poor skin integrity R/T immobility from hip fracture

24. What is the priority factor in establishing a plan of care for a patient who will be on a routine antihypertensive medication at home?

    a. Patient education on adverse effects of the medication

    b. Risk for noncompliance

    c. Arranging for the drug to be delivered

    d. Teaching the patient to take own blood pressure

25. What factor established from the patient's health history would most likely suggest noncompliance with the medication regimen?

    a. Male

    b. Female

    c. Elderly

    d. Live in a rural area

26. When the nurse educates a patient with special needs, which of the following would be appropriate?

    a. Use of special education tools

    b. Use of medical terminology

    c. No patient education required

    d. Assigning the task to someone else

MAKING CONNECTIONS

27. All drugs have more than one:

    a. Name

    b. Active ingredient

    c. Generic name

    d. Indication

28. How do therapeutic drugs differ from foods, household products, and cosmetics?

    a. Only therapeutic drugs can induce a biologic response.

    b. Food, household products, and cosmetics are not traditionally designed for the treatment of disease and suffering.

    c. Drugs may not be considered part of the body's normal activities.

    d. Drugs are narrowly defined.

29. Which method is used for fast delivery of a drug to the cerebral spinal fluid?

    a. Intraperitoneal

    b. Intrathecal

    c. Epidural

    d. Transmucosal

30. Which term describes how much of a drug is available to produce a biologic response?

    a. Volume of distribution

    b. Rate of elimination

    c. Bioavailability

    d. Half-life

31. What is the process of moving a drug from its site of administration across one or more body membranes called?

    a. Absorption

    b. Metabolism

    c. Distribution

    d. Excretion

CASE STUDY APPLICATIONS

32. Ms. P is 15 years old and has just been diagnosed with type 1 diabetes mellitus. She has presented to the emergency department on three occasions with blood glucose of over 400. She refuses to follow her prescribed diet and insulin regimen. She states, "My friends and classmates think that I am weird when I don't eat what they do and when I have to give myself a shot." As the nurse, you must remember certain factors related to this age group when establishing your plan of care.

    a. What is the self-image focus at this age?

    b. Would you consider this a special consideration patient in regard to patient education?

    c. What would be your priority nursing diagnosis?

33. Mrs. G is a 35-year-old Hispanic migrant worker who does not speak or understand English. She presents to the emergency department with severe abdominal pain and rigidity in the right lower quadrant. As the nurse in charge, you are to take the health history and establish a plan of care.

    a. What would be your priority intervention in this patient's plan of care?

    b. What barriers would you expect to encounter when establishing her plan of care?

34. Mr. W is a 25-year-old patient with a history of substance abuse. He has been admitted to your area after receiving critical injuries in a car wreck. He is now recovering and has moved to the acute ward from ICU. As the nurse establishing his plan of care, you may encounter barriers in regard to his recovery.

    a. What effect will his substance abuse have on his recovery?

    b. What goals and outcomes will you establish for this patient?

CHAPTER 9

LEGAL AND ETHICAL ISSUES RELATED TO DRUG ADMINISTRATION

OBJECTIVES

To view the objectives, please refer to the textbook, student CD-ROM, and the Companion Website at *www.prenhall.com/adams*.

FILL IN THE BLANK

From the textbook, find the correct word(s) to complete the statement(s).

1. The _____ Act governs the qualifications and competencies of all nurses, state by state, in order to _____.

2. Nursing ethics are judged on the moral principles of _____, _____, _____, _____, _____, and _____.

3. Legal issues are compared to what a _____ and _____ nurse would do.

4. The steps of the Nursing Process are _____, _____, _____, and _____.

5. If a nursing intervention is not _____ it is not considered as being done.

6. The five rights of medication administration are _____, _____, _____, _____, and _____.

7. An ethical dilemma occurs when two moral _____ are in _____.

8. A medication error is any _____ event that may cause or lead to inappropriate drug use or cause _____ harm while the medication is in the control of the nurse, patient, or consumer.

9. Incomplete orders should be _____ with the prescriber before the drug is _____.

10. It is the nurses _____ and _____ responsibility to report any and all medication errors.

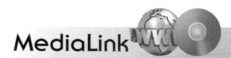

MATCHING

For questions 11 through 17, match the term in column I with the correct definition in column II.

Column I	Column II
11. _____ Beneficence	a. Patient has a right to refuse medications
12. _____ Maleficence	b. Nurse must seek to do good for the patient
13. _____ Autonomy	c. Moral principles that guide decision making
14. _____ Veracity	d. Nurse is obliged to fulfill promises to patient
15. _____ Justice	e. Patient expects the nurse to do the patient no harm
16. _____ Fidelity	f. Nurse is obliged to be fair to all patients
17. _____ Ethics	g. Patient expects the nurse to be truthful

MULTIPLE CHOICE

18. The ANA Code of Ethics addresses all of the following except:

    a. Respect for human dignity

    b. Patient's right to privacy

    c. Standards of nursing practice

    d. Criteria for licensure

19. What best describes moral principles guiding ethical nursing practice?

    a. Personal and individualized

    b. Common to all cultures

    c. Only affect the terminally ill

    d. Best utilized for accident victims

20. Nurse practice acts differ from state to state but have which of the following in common?

    a. Definition of professional nursing

    b. Who may administer medications

    c. Safe delivery of medications

    d. All of the above

21. Assessment is the most important step of the Nursing Process in preventing medication errors by which of the following?

    a. Having the patient state the outcome of the medication

    b. Obtaining allergy and medication history information

    c. Advising the patient to question the nurse about medications

    d. Planning the correct times for the patient to take medications

22. Documentation of medication requires that a drug should be which of the following?

    a. Given before it is documented

    b. Documented first and then given

   c. Checked against previous orders

   d. Not documented if refused by the patient

23. Which best describes medication errors?

   a. Always preventable events

   b. Intentional adverse events

   c. Not preventable events

   d. Reportable events

24. Which best describes the reporting of medication errors?

   a. Is voluntary in ethical nursing practice

   b. Must be kept confidential in nursing practice

   c. Is an optional act on the part of the nurse

   d. Is responsible and accountable by the nurse

25. Which best describes incident reports?

   a. Initiated by the nurse who identifies the error

   b. Initiated by the nurse who commits the error

   c. Valued in performance evaluations

   d. Kept in confidence by quality assurance

26. Preventing medication errors is the goal of whom?

   a. Every nurse

   b. All nurses

   c. Every consumer

   d. All of the above

27. State law refers to which of the following?

   a. What a nurse "must do" according to the Nurse Practice Act

   b. What a nurse "ought to do" according to the Code of Ethics

   c. Reasonable and prudent actions in all spheres of life

   d. None of the above

MAKING CONNECTIONS

28. Which federal agency is responsible for determining the effectiveness of all new drugs proposed each year?

   a. Federal Drug Administration (FDA)

   b. Drug Enforcement Agency (DEA)

   c. National Institute for Health (NIH)

   d. United States Public Health Service (USPHS)

29. All narcotics are assigned a schedule or classification by law. In which schedule will you find morphine sulfate?

    a. Schedule I

    b. Schedule II

    c. Schedule III

    d. Schedule IV

30. What does it mean when a drug is classified as being teratogenic?

    a. It is safe for the mother in the first trimester of pregnancy.

    b. It is safe for the mother in the last trimester of pregnancy.

    c. Harmful effects on the fetus may occur at high doses.

    d. It is not safe for fetus and will cause abnormalities if given.

31. Which of the following parenteral routes of medication administration is primarily used for diagnostic purposes?

    a. Intramuscular injection

    b. Intrathecal injection

    c. Subcutaneous injection

    d. Intradermal injection

32. Which legal agency deals with the enforcement of substance abuse laws?

    a. Federal Drug Administration (FDA)

    b. Drug Enforcement Agency (DEA)

    c. National Institute for Health (NIH)

    d. None of the above

CASE STUDY APPLICATIONS

33. An elderly patient refuses an antihypertensive drug after breakfast. You note that this has happened 3 days in a row. The patient's blood pressure has risen 40 mm Hg and the patient complains of an occipital headache.

    a. What step of the Nursing Process is utilized in this scenario? What type of data is described in this process?

    b. In developing your plan of care for this patient, what ethical principle would you include in your interventions?

34. While you are administering medications to your patient, you note that she has the same medications at the bedside in opened containers.

    a. What would be your short-term goal for this patient?

    b. What evaluation criteria would you utilize in evaluating this goal?

35. While you are preparing drugs for your patient, you note that he has been receiving an anticoagulant daily but the order reads to be given every other day.

    a. What would be an appropriate nursing diagnosis for this patient?

    b. What nursing interventions would be included in the plan of care?

CHAPTER 10

BIOSOCIAL ASPECTS OF PHARMACOTHERAPY

OBJECTIVES

To view the objectives, please refer to the textbook, student CD-ROM, and the Companion Website at *www.prenhall.com/adams*.

FILL IN THE BLANK

From the textbook, find the correct word(s) to complete the statement(s).

1. The recipient of care must be regarded in a _____ context for health to be impacted in a positive manner.

2. Strong spiritual or religious beliefs may greatly influence a person's _____ of illness and the _____ of treatment.

3. Culturally competent nursing requires knowledge of the _____, _____, and _____ of various people.

4. The most obvious community-related influence on pharmacotherapy is _____ to healthcare.

5. Antihypertensive agents used in men may cause _____.

6. An issue of gender inequity regarding prescription drug coverage for women is that _____ have been excluded from coverage.

7. _____ and _____ are disciplines founded on objective, logical, and critical deliberation.

8. _____ and _____ are disciplines based on intuitive and subjective considerations.

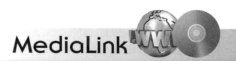

MediaLink

www.prenhall.com/adams

CD-ROM
Audio Glossary
NCLEX Review

Companion Website
NCLEX Review
Case Study
Expanded Key Concepts
Challenge Your Knowledge

MATCHING

For questions 9 through 15, match the definition in column I with its key term in column II.

Column I	Column II
9. _____ Change in enzyme structure and function due to mutation in DNA	a. Culture
	b. Ethnic
10. _____ Science that deals with normal and abnormal processes and their impact on behavior	c. Genetic polymorphism
	d. Holistic
11. _____ Study of human behavior within the context of groups and societies	e. Psychology
	f. Sociology
12. _____ Incorporates the capacity to love, to convey compassion, to enjoy life, and to find peace of mind and fulfillment	g. Spirituality
13. _____ Community of people having a common history and similar genetic heritage	
14. _____ Beliefs, values, customs, and religious rituals shared by a group of people	
15. _____ Each person viewed as an integrated whole	

MULTIPLE CHOICE

16. The patient's psychosocial history is essential in the initial assessment. It includes all of the following except:

   a. Religious beliefs

   b. Sexual practices

   c. Previous illnesses

   d. Use of alcohol, tobacco, or illegal drugs

17. Which of the following patients is least likely to be compliant with a medication regimen?

   a. The patient who trusts the nurse

   b. The patient who is aware of possible severe side effects associated with medications

   c. The patient who has high expectations regarding the results of taking medications

   d. The patient who has received limited information about medications

18. Which of the following people is least likely to encounter obstacles when seeking healthcare?

   a. Single mother with four children who lives in the inner city

   b. Family with four children who live in a rural area

   c. Elderly patient on a fixed income

   d. Suburban housewife

19. Community-related variables that influence pharmacotherapy include all except:

   a. Access to healthcare

   b. Alternative therapies

c. Literacy

d. Spiritual beliefs

20. Which of the following statements by the nurse will ensure that the patient understands the instructions given?

    a. "Mrs. Johnson, do you understand how to take your meds?"

    b. "Mrs. Johnson, you take this drug at 8 A.M. and 8 P.M. Call the doctor if you have any problems."

    c. "Mrs. Johnson, could you explain to me how you will take your medication at home?"

    d. "Mrs. Johnson here are some printed instructions on how to use your prescription meds."

21. What is the study of changes in enzyme structure and function caused by mutations in DNA called?

    a. Pharmacogenetics

    b. Eugenics

    c. Polymorphisms

    d. Acetylation

22. Which of the following drugs would have the least effect on a person of African American descent, due to enzyme polymorphisms?

    a. Isoniazid

    b. Propranolol

    c. Codeine

    d. Procainamide

23. Which of the following statements regarding women's health is false?

    a. Women seek healthcare earlier than men.

    b. Women have a higher incidence of Alzheimer's disease than men.

    c. Women do not seek medical attention for potential cardiac problems as readily as men.

    d. Women do not like to use antihypertensive medications due to side effects.

24. Variables to consider when treating patients in different ethnic groups include all except:

    a. Diet

    b. Alternative therapies

    c. Genetic differences

    d. Literacy

25. Which of the following is the least useful method for supplying information regarding medication use at home to a patient who is functionally illiterate?

    a. Provide the patient with typewritten information regarding the drug and its side effects.

    b. Provide the patient with diagrams and pictures showing how to use the inhaler.

    c. Instruct the patient's family about the inhaler at the same time the patient is receiving the information.

    d. Show the patient the inhaler each time it is administered and explain its use and side effects.

MAKING CONNECTIONS

26. Which of the following choices distinguishes a traditional drug from a biologic or natural alternative agent? A traditional drug is:

    a. Used routinely by nurses

    b. An extract from a natural source

    c. Produced in very small amounts

    d. Accepted by most religions in the United States

27. Which of the following drug schedules has the highest potential for abuse?

    a. Schedule I

    b. Schedule II

    c. Schedule III

    d. Schedule IV

28. Which of the following diseases may be delivered by bioterrorists using ultrafine powder?

    a. Smallpox

    b. Anthrax

    c. Plague

    d. Polio

29. Ms. Thomas is in her first trimester of pregnancy. She has been told not to use a drug the physician called "teratogenic." She asks you what this term means. You tell her it is a substance:

    a. That could produce dependency

    b. That will harm her developing fetus

    c. Used to induce labor

    d. That cannot be obtained over the counter

30. Which of the following drug delivery methods is not a parenteral method of drug delivery, and avoids the first-pass effect in the liver?

    a. Oral

    b. Intrathecal

    c. Intramuscular

    d. Sublingual

CASE STUDY APPLICATIONS

31. Mrs. J has come in for her monthly prenatal checkup. During your assessment she confides that her husband is an alcoholic. His parents were both alcoholics, as well. Mrs. J tearfully asks you whether this is a genetic condition, and what are the chances her child will have a problem with alcohol abuse.

    a. What other assessments must you make?

    b. How will you answer her question?

    c. What other interventions might you include in your care plan for helping Mrs. J deal with this situation?

32. Mr. F, age 50, has been admitted to the hospital with a diagnosis of accelerated hypertension. He informs you he quit taking his medications several weeks ago. During your initial assessment you determine that Mr. F has excellent prescription drug insurance coverage.

    a. What other factors related to use of his medications must be assessed in this situation?

    b. You determine that Mr. F has little knowledge regarding his medications, and plan patient teaching as one of your primary nursing interventions. What information do you need to give Mr. F regarding the use of his antihypertensives?

33. Ms. L has been admitted to your floor with multiple compression fractures of her lumbar vertebrae. On your initial assessment she is obviously in pain—her face is pale, diaphoretic, and drawn. She is gripping the side rail with her hand. When you offer her a narcotic for pain relief she refuses, saying, "It's not God's will for us to use medicines that cloud the mind so that we can't think about His goodness to us."

    a. What other modes of treatment could you include in your care plan that Ms. L might find more compatible with her religious beliefs?

    b. What other assessments should you make on Ms. L in order to help her further?

    c. Are there any medications she might be willing to consider if you offered them?

CHAPTER 11

HERBAL AND ALTERNATIVE THERAPIES

OBJECTIVES

To view the objectives, please refer to the text book, student CD-ROM, and the Companion Website at *www.prenhall.com/adams*.

FILL IN THE BLANK

From the text book, find the correct word(s) to complete the statement(s).

1. Many people think the advantage of natural substances over synthetic medications is that they have more _____.

2. From the perspective of pharmacology, the value of CAM therapies lies in their ability to _____ the need for _____.

3. The nurse should not be _____ when the patient requests alternative treatment.

4. An herb is technically a botanical without any _____ such as _____ or _____.

5. When collecting herbs for use at home it is essential to know which portion of the plant contains the _____.

6. Herbs may contain _____ of active chemicals, many of which have not been isolated, studied, or even _____.

7. Herbal products are regulated by the _____ Act.

MATCHING

For questions 8 through 12, match the description in column I with its formulation in column II.

Column I	Column II
8. _____ Extraction of active ingredients using organic solvents to form a highly concentrated liquid or solid	a. Tea
	b. Infusion

9. _____ Fresh or dried herbs soaked in hot
water for at least 15 minutes

10. _____ Fresh or dried herbs are soaked in hot
water for 5 to 10 minutes before
ingestion

11. _____ Fresh or dried herbs are boiled in
water for 30 to 60 minutes until most
water has boiled off

12. _____ Herb is soaked in alcohol which
remains as part of the liquid

c. Decoction

d. Tincture

e. Extract

For questions 13 through 22, match the example in column I with the therapy name in column II.

Column I	**Column II**
13. _____ Faith and prayer	a. Biological-based therapy
14. _____ Yoga	b. Alternate healthcare systems
15. _____ Biofeedback	c. Manual healing
16. _____ Nutritional supplements	d. Mind-body interventions
17. _____ Homeopathy	e. Spiritual
18. _____ Acupuncture, Chinese herbs	
19. _____ Chiropractic	
20. _____ Music, dance	
21. _____ Shamans	
22. _____ Massage	

MULTIPLE CHOICE

23. Common characteristics of complimentary and alternative medicine (CAM) systems include all of the following except:

a. They consider the health of the whole person

b. They promote disease prevention, self-care, and self-healing

c. They recognize the role of spirituality in health and healing

d. They provide inexpensive supplements and substitutes for expensive traditional drugs

24. With the rising of the pharmaceutical industry in the late 1800s, interest in herbal medicine began to wane because of what reason?

a. Herbs became very expensive.

b. Herbs were no longer readily available in the environment.

c. Synthetic drugs could be standardized and produced more cheaply.

d. Herbs were proven to be ineffective against most diseases.

25. Which of the following is *not* a major factor contributing to the recent increase in popularity of botanicals?

    a. Many herbs have been clearly demonstrated to be more effective than available drugs.

    b. Herbal products are more widely available to the public.

    c. The herbal industry has aggressively marketed its products.

    d. Herbal products cost considerably less than most prescription medicines.

26. Which of the following statements regarding herbs is false?

    a. Herbs may contain dozens of active chemicals.

    b. The chemicals in herbs may not have the same activity if they are isolated from each other.

    c. Herbal preparations are standardized and the exact quantities of active chemicals are known.

    d. The strength of an herbal preparation may vary depending upon where it was grown and how it was stored.

27. Products intended to enhance the diet such as botanicals, vitamins, minerals, or any other extract or metabolite that is not already approved as a drug by the FDA are defined as which of the following?

    a. Herbal products

    b. Alternative therapies

    c. Supplemental therapies

    d. Dietary supplements

28. Which of the following is a legal requirement contained in the DSHEA?

    a. Dietary supplements must be tested for safety prior to marketing.

    b. Efficacy must be demonstrated by the manufacturer.

    c. The herbal product must contain only one active ingredient.

    d. Dietary supplements must state that the product is not intended to diagnose, treat, cure, or prevent any disease.

29. Which of the following statements would most likely *not* be allowed on the label of a dietary supplement?

    a. Helps promote a healthy immune system

    b. May reduce pain and inflammation

    c. Reduces blood pressure and the risk of stroke

    d. May improve cardiovascular function

30. What responsibility does the healthcare provider have in regard to herbal products?

    a. Seek to dissuade the client from using them because they are not "scientific"

    b. Be aware of the latest medical information on herbal products including interactions and side effects

    c. Inform clients that they can trust the labeling on herbal products because the U.S. government has a rigorous testing program before the product is marketed

    d. Tell the client to seek information on herbal products from a practitioner of alternative medicine rather than a physician, because the physician has no knowledge of these products

31. Which popular herb is used for its possible benefit in treating depression?

    a. Aloe

b. Astragalus

c. St. John's wort

d. Ginger

32. Which popular herb is used for its possible beneficial effect on the immune system?

    a. Black cohosh

    b. Echinacea

    c. Ginkgo

    d. Kava kava

33. Saw palmetto is a popular herb that is taken for what potential effect?

    a. Relief of urinary problems related to enlarged prostate

    b. Reduction of stress and to promote sleep

    c. Reduction of blood cholesterol levels

    d. Treatment of constipation

34. Mrs. Baxter is an insulin-dependent diabetic. She has come to the doctor complaining of frequent hypoglycemic episodes. She tells you she is taking all of the following dietary supplements. Which one needs to be considered as a possible cause of her hypoglycemia?

    a. Ginger

    b. Ginkgo biloba

    c. Echinacea

    d. Garlic

MAKING CONNECTIONS

35. Which of the following choices distinguishes a conventional drug from a natural alternative agent?

    a. A natural alternative agent is obtained from a natural source.

    b. A conventional drug is routinely used by healthcare providers.

    c. A conventional drug is chemically produced.

    d. A natural alternative must be tested by the FDA.

36. Which of the following statements best describes an advantage of prescription drugs over OTC drugs?

    a. OTC drugs do not require a physician's order.

    b. Prescription drugs ensure that harmful reactions, ineffective treatment, or a progressive disease state will not occur.

    c. Only clients authorized to receive prescription drugs will take these medications.

    d. The healthcare provider can maximize therapy by ordering the amount and frequency to be dispensed.

37. Why might rectal drugs be administered to a client?

   a. The client is unconscious.

   b. The client is experiencing nausea or vomiting.

   c. The client is an infant who cannot swallow pills.

   d. All of the above are correct.

38. Which of the following drug administration methods is used when rapid results are required?

   a. Intravenous

   b. Intramuscular

   c. Oral

   d. Rectal

39. The client who is most likely to benefit from a prescription drug is the one who:

   a. Has prescription drug coverage through an insurance company

   b. Sees the physician regularly and follows the directions for using the drug

   c. Is not aware that the drug can cause serious side effects

   d. Uses herbal supplements and goes to the doctor only when these fail to work

CASE STUDY APPLICATIONS

40. Mr. S, age 78, is being discharged from your unit on Lanoxin and Coumadin. Your care plan includes patient education regarding these drugs. You have included his wife in the teaching session, and she mentions that she believes his problems can be corrected by using naturally grown herbs rather than drugs. Mr. S states, "I'm going to do what the doctor says, but a few weeds can't hurt me. I'll take them to keep her happy."

   a. What further assessments are indicated in this situation?

   b. Your care plan has been altered to give additional information on herbal preparations to this couple. What information must you give to Mr. and Mrs. S regarding the use of herbs while on Coumadin and Lanoxin?

   c. What other information regarding the use of herbal products should be given to this patient?

41. Mrs. R comes to your mental health outpatient clinic with new symptoms, including agitation, headache, and dizziness. You note on assessment that she is also profusely diaphoretic. Mrs. R has been treated for depression with Prozac, an SSRI. During your assessment she confides that she has been using St. John's wort with her prescription drugs. She asks if her prescription can be changed to something that "works better."

   a. What is a likely cause of Mrs. R's symptoms?

   b. Your initial plan of care is for patient education regarding drug-herb interactions. What other antidepressants might interact unfavorably with St. John's wort?

42. Mr. K, a 42-year-old teacher, has been using echinacea regularly, yet he now has the flu. During your assessment you note that he has rheumatoid arthritis, for which he is taking methotrexate. He is upset that he has become ill, and feels that the advertisements in nutrition magazines and on television may have misled him into buying useless products. He asks your advice regarding the value of alternative therapies.

   a. Your nursing interventions call for monitoring specific lab values in view of Mr. K's use of echinacea and methotrexate. Which lab values would you monitor, and why?

   b. Your care plan includes patient education regarding the uses of alternative therapies. What information should be included?

   c. During team conference, a colleague suggests that a goal for Mr. K's care should be "discontinues use of all supplements and uses only prescription drugs." Tell why you disagree with her suggestion, and write an improved goal.

CHAPTER 12

SUBSTANCE ABUSE

OBJECTIVES

To view the objectives, please refer to the textbook, student CD-ROM, and the Companion Website at *www.prenhall.com/adams*.

FILL IN THE BLANK

From the textbook, find the correct word(s) to complete the statement(s).

1. The most commonly abused drugs are _____ and _____.

2. Three substances that come from natural sources and are frequently abused are _____, _____, and _____.

3. The risk of addiction to prescription drugs is based on _____ and _____.

4. Two categories used to classify substance dependence are _____ and _____.

5. _____ is when a person has an overwhelming desire to take a drug and cannot stop.

6. Psychological dependence may develop after one dose of _____.

7. It is common to treat alcohol withdrawal with a short-acting _____.

8. Opioid withdrawal can be treated with _____.

9. After several months of pain therapy, a patient must increase the dose of the pain medication. The best description of this situation is that the patient has developed _____ for the pain medication.

10. All hallucinogenic drugs are Schedule _____ drugs.

11. _____ is a drug often applied via transdermal patch to ease signs of drug discontinuation including agitation, weight gain, anxiety, headache, and an extreme craving.

12. Signs of physical discomfort after drug use is discontinued are referred to as classic _____ symptoms.

MATCHING

For questions 13 through 20, match the drug or substance in column I with its group name in column II.

Column I	**Column II**
13. _____ Lysergic acid diethylamide (LSD)	a. Hallucinogen
14. _____ Pentobarbital (Nembutal)	b. CNS stimulant
15. _____ Alprazolam (Xanax)	c. CNS depressant
16. _____ Methadone (Dolophine)	d. Opioid
17. _____ Dextroamphetamine (Dexedrine)	
18. _____ Methylphenidate (Ritalin)	
19. _____ Propoxyphene (Darvon)	
20. _____ MDMA (Ecstasy)	

For questions 21 through 25, match the symptoms of withdrawal in column I with their drug classification in column II.

Column I	**Column II**
21. _____ Depression	a. Opioid
22. _____ Dilated pupils	b. Nicotine
23. _____ Goose bumps	c. Cocaine
24. _____ Increased appetite	
25. _____ Yawning	

For questions 26 through 29, match the drug/substance in column I with its source in column II.

Column I	**Column II**
26. _____ Opium	a. Natural
27. _____ MDMA	b. Synthetic
28. _____ Cocaine	
29. _____ LSD	

MULTIPLE CHOICE

30. All abused substances affect which body system?

    a. Cardiovascular

    b. Nervous

    c. Digestive

    d. Respiratory

31. You are working with a patient who has a diagnosis of alcoholism. What organ system is most likely to be malfunctioning for this patient?

    a. Lungs

    b. Bowels

c. Liver

d. Kidneys

32. A patient is admitted with liver failure. What nursing action is most appropriate prior to delivery of medications for this patient?

   a. Check drug dosing because of issues related to metabolism.

   b. Request increase in blood clotting drugs because of liver dysfunction.

   c. Hold all nutritional supplements until liver disease is resolved.

   d. Expect increase in drug dosing of antibiotics because of immune compromise.

33. Repeated use of caffeine products can create which of the following effects?

   a. Decreased stomach acid

   b. Decreased blood pressure

   c. Increased fatigue

   d. Increased urination

34. What drug was once used for bronchodilation but has been discontinued because of psychotic episodes in some patients?

   a. Cocaine

   b. LSD

   c. Phencyclidine

   d. Amphetamine

35. Which of the following statements about addiction is *not* correct?

   a. Addiction is most likely a neurobiological problem linked closely to the patient's psychological state and social setting.

   b. In some cases, addiction may begin with the patient's medical need for the treatment of an illness.

   c. The therapeutic use of narcotics and sedatives creates large numbers of addicted patients.

   d. Attempts to predict a patient's addictive tendency using psychological profiles or genetic markers has largely been unsuccessful.

36. Which of the following drugs was once used as a local anesthetic?

   a. Amphetamine

   b. Ketamine

   c. Phencyclidine

   d. Cocaine

37. What is the term for when a person has an overwhelming desire to take a drug and cannot stop?

    a. Addiction

    b. Dependence

    c. Tolerance

    d. Withdrawal

38. What term describes when an individual adapts to a drug over a short time and requires higher and higher doses to produce the same effect?

    a. Conditioning

    b. Withdrawal

    c. Immunity

    d. Tolerance

39. What is the sleep disorder drug class for which patients often fake or change prescriptions?

    a. Amphetamines

    b. Barbiturates

    c. Benzodiazepines

    d. Opioids

CASE STUDY APPLICATIONS

40. A 28-year-old patient is admitted to the hospital with pneumonia. During your assessment of the social history, you learn the patient has a job, is self-reliant, and smokes marijuana every other night, but does not drink alcohol. The patient claims "smoking a joint now and then doesn't hurt anybody."

    a. Based on your understanding of marijuana, what would you teach this patient regarding the long-term effects of marijuana?

    b. Describe the psychological effects of marijuana and explain how dependence might develop in this case.

    c. Compare the marijuana risks to those of smoking tobacco products.

41. A patient admitted for recurrent bladder infections describes a 15-year history of drinking beer and wine in moderate amounts. The patient gives a family history of paternal alcoholism. The patient asks, "What kinds of factors are linked with addiction? Is it genetic, or is there some other reason why people become addicted?"

    a. What would you include in the teaching plan to answer the patient's questions?

    b. What assessment data are important when you admit this patient?

    c. What nursing diagnoses and what patient outcomes would you write?

CHAPTER 13

DRUGS AFFECTING THE AUTONOMIC NERVOUS SYSTEM

OBJECTIVES

To view the objectives, please refer to the textbook, student CD-Rom, and the Companion Website at *www.prenhall.com/adams*.

FILL IN THE BLANK

From the textbook, find the correct word(s) to complete the statement(s).

1. The two primary divisions of the nervous system are the

   _____ nervous system, made up of the brain and

   spinal cord, and the _____ nervous system.

2. The _____ nervous system provides involuntary control over smooth muscle, cardiac muscle, and glands.

3. The sympathetic nervous system produces the _____ response; the parasympathetic nervous

   system produces symptoms called the _____ response.

4. According to the textbook, three parts of a synapse are the _____ nerve, the _____, and

   the _____ nerve.

5. _____ is the main neurotransmitter responsible for sympathetic nervous transmission;

   _____ is the main neurotransmitter responsible for parasympathetic nervous transmission.

6. Sympathetic nerves are often called _____, a term coming from the word *adrenaline*;

   parasympathetic nerves are called _____.

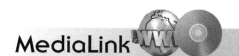

MediaLink

www.prenhall.com/adams

CD-ROM
Audio Glossary
NCLEX Review

Companion Website
NCLEX Review
Case Study
Expanded Key Concepts

7. Increased heart rate, bronchodilation, decreased motility in the GI tract, mydriasis, and decreased secretions from glands are physiologic responses associated with inactivation of the _____ nervous system or activation of the _____ nervous system.

8. _____ blockers, primarily used for hypertension, comprise the most commonly prescribed autonomic medications.

9. A class of drugs named after the fight-or-flight response and primarily used for increasing the heart rate, dilating the bronchi, and drying secretions resulting from colds is _____ drugs.

10. _____ drugs, named after the rest-and-digest response, are commonly used to stimulate the urinary or digestive tracts following general anesthesia.

MATCHING

For questions 11 through 15, match the physiologic responses in column I with the autonomic receptor classes in column II.

Column I

11. _____ Cause dry mouth, constipation, urinary retention, and increased heart rate

12. _____ Relax vascular smooth muscle and dry nasal secretions

13. _____ Cause bronchodilation

14. ——— Lower blood pressure without affecting the heart

15. _____ Decrease heart rate

Column II

a. $Beta_1$-blockers

b. $Alpha_1$-blockers

c. $Beta_2$-agonists

d. $Alpha_2$-agonists

e. Cholinergic (muscarinic) blockers

For questions 16 through 20, match the peripheral nervous system drug in column I with the indication in column II.

Column I

16. _____ Atropine (Isopto Atropine)

17. _____ Bethanechol (Urecholine)

18. _____ Pyridostigmine (Mestinon)

19. ——— Doxazosin (Cardura)

20. _____ Albuterol (Proventil)

Column II

a. Myasthenia gravis

b. GI stimulation following surgery

c. Pupil dilation during an eye exam

d. Asthma inhaler

e. Hypertension

For questions 21 through 25, match the drug in column I with the classification in column II.

Column I

21. _____ Scopolamine (Hyoscine)

22. _____ Phenylephrine (Neo-Synephrine)

23. _____ Bethanechol (Urecholine)

24. _____ Propranolol (Inderal)

25. _____ Dobutamine (Dobutrex)

Column II

a. Parasympathomimetic

b. Anticholinergic

c. Sympathomimetic

d. Adrenergic blocker

MULTIPLE CHOICE

26. A patient is discharged with a newly prescribed antagonist for control of hypertension. The nurse gives discharge instructions. It is inappropriate to include which of the following instructions prior to the patient's leaving?

    a. Report any difficulty with urination to the nurse.

    b. Take the medication for the first time directly prior to getting into bed.

    c. Monitor BP and pulse daily, giving parameters that need to be reported.

    d. Return for lab tests to monitor renal function.

27. An adrenergic blocker is *most directly* related to which of the following?

    a. Stimulation of the sympathetic nervous system

    b. Inhibition of the parasympathetic nervous system

    c. Stimulation of the parasympathetic nervous system

    d. Inhibition of the sympathetic nervous system

28. How does bethanechol (Urecholine) exert its effects?

    a. Stimulates cholinergic receptors

    b. Blocks cholinergic receptors

    c. Blocks beta-receptors

    d. Stimulates alpha-receptors

29. What drugs block the action of norepinephrine at alpha- and beta-receptors?

    a. Parasympathomimetics

    b. Parasympatholytics

    c. Sympathomimetics

    d. Sympatholytics

30. A nurse is to give phenylephrine parenterally. What safety precaution would be necessary especially with this drug?

    a. Monitor patency throughout the infusion.

    b. Monitor temp of patient q1h during the infusion.

    c. Monitor for CNS depression.

    d. Monitor for hypotension throughout the infusion.

31. Parasympathomimetics are safe for patients diagnosed with which of the following?

    a. Myasthenia gravis

    b. GI obstruction

    c. Asthma

    d. Angina or dysrhythmias

32. How does propanolol (Inderal) exert its effects?

    a. Stimulates cholinergic receptors

    b. Blocks cholinergic receptors

    c. Blocks beta-receptors

    d. Stimulates alpha-receptors

33. Pseudoephedrine has been ordered for a patient with nasal congestion. The nurse knows the drug can give which of the following side effects?

    a. Hypertension, insomnia, and tachycardia

    b. Drowsiness and dry mouth

    c. Increased heart rate and abdominal cramps

    d. Dilated pupils and orthostatic hypotension

34. Anticholinergics may be used in treatment of peptic ulcers. What action makes this drug useful in this condition?

    a. Decreases gastric emptying time

    b. Decreases gastric acid secretions

    c. Decreases intestinal motility

    d. Relaxes gastric smooth muscles

35. What are sympathomimetics also called?

    a. Cholinergic agonists

    b. Adrenergic agonists

    c. Cholinergic blockers

    d. Adrenergic blockers

36. Epinephrine is a nonselective adrenergic agonist. What is the disadvantage of this nonspecific action?

    a. It causes more autonomic side effects.

    b. This drug cannot be used for nervous system conditions.

    c. It will not cross the blood-brain barrier.

    d. It can only be given by SC injection.

37. A patient is prescribed Mestinon for myasthenia gravis. Which of the following would be inappropriate to teach the patient?

    a. Take the drug at the same times each day.

    b. Take drug on a full stomach.

    c. Monitor liver enzymes as requested.

    d. Maintain a journal of episodes of weakness and how long it occurs after the drug is given.

38. Neostigmine is an example of which of the following?

    a. Cholinergic blocker

    b. Nicotinic blocker

    c. Cholinergic agonist

    d. Cholinesterase inhibitor

39. Which of the following drugs would dry up body secretions?

    a. Bethanechol (Urecholine)

    b. Metoprolol (Lopressor)

    c. Atropine (Isopto Atropine)

    d. Doxazosin (Cardura)

40. Atropine is usually not prescribed for any patient with glaucoma. The nurse knows the contraindication is due to which of the following effects of atropine?

    a. Increase in intraocular pressure

    b. Decrease in lacrimation

    c. Decrease in lateral movement of the eyes

    d. Increase in difficulty with night vision due to papillary constriction

MAKING CONNECTIONS

41. Methylphenidate (Ritalin) is most similar to which abused substance?

    a. Tetrahydrocannabinol (THC)

    b. Ketamine

    c. Methamphetamine

    d. Ethyl alcohol

42. When a drug is referred to as an agonist, it can do which of the following?

    a. Be a facilitator of an action

    b. Be an inhibitor of an action

    c. Have a potentiated action

    d. Make one drug interact with another drug

43. What are the most commonly abused sympathomimetics?

    a. Amphetamines

    b. Proventil

    c. Sudafed/pseudoephedrine

    d. Marijuana

44. What is an example of an illegal CNS stimulant?

    a. Propoxyphene (Darvon)

    b. Flurazepam (Dalmane)

    c. Heroin

    d. Cocaine

45. The nurse is to administer medications using the "five rights." To give medications to a patient without an ID bracelet violates which of the rights?

    a. Right medications

    b. Right time

    c. Right patient

    d. Right route

CALCULATIONS

46. The physician orders metaproterenol sulfate 20 mg qid. The pharmacy sends metaproterenol syrup 10 mg/5 cc. The patient should receive _____cc per day.

47. The physician orders 0.3 mg atropine sulfate SC q4h. The pharmacy sends atropine sulfate 0.6 mg/ml. The nurse should administer _____ml SC q4h.

CASE STUDY APPLICATIONS

48. Mr. Z, age 80, has been diagnosed with COPD and hypertension. The patient has been given propranolol (Inderal) to treat the hypertension. The nurse is assessing the following medications that he is also taking.

    Benadryl 25 mg q4h for itching and sneezing due to allergies

    Prazosin bid for hypertension

    Proventil inhaler PRN for wheezing

    a. Identify three potential nursing diagnoses that could occur due to drug interactions when these medications are given concurrently. Explain why these interactions would occur.

    b. What nursing interventions can be done to decrease the risk of the problems created with these interactions?

49. Ms. W, diagnosed with myasthenia gravis, comes to the ER with muscle weakness. The nurse, during the history, determines that the patient has been taking double doses of her pyradostigmine (Mestinon) over the past several days.

    a. What assessment would the nurse make to identify a nursing diagnosis?

    b. What nursing diagnosis would you identify?

    c. What nursing interventions could be used in the above diagnosis?

CHAPTER 14

DRUGS FOR ANXIETY AND INSOMNIA

OBJECTIVES

To view the objectives, please refer to the textbook, student CD-ROM, and the Companion Website at *www.prenhall.com/adams*.

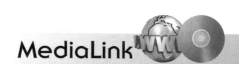

MediaLink www.prenhall.com/adams

CD-ROM
Audio Glossary
NCLEX Review

Companion Website
NCLEX Review
Dosage Calculations
Care Plans
Expanded Key Concepts

FILL IN THE BLANK

From the textbook, find the correct word(s) to complete the statement(s).

1. Apprehension, tension, or uneasiness lasting for 6 months or longer and causing considerable stress is referred to as _____.

2. Two important sets of brain structures are associated with anxiety. One connected with emotion is the _____ system; the other, projecting from the brainstem and connected with alertness, is the _____ system.

3. _____ are classes of drugs prescribed to relax patients. Classes of drugs used to help patients to sleep are _____.

4. Diazepam (Valium) reduces anxiety by binding to a receptor in the brain referred to as the _____ channel molecule.

5. The drug class usually prescribed for short-term insomnia caused by anxiety is _____.

6. _____ is a class of drugs that reduces anxiety, causes drowsiness, and promotes sleep when administered at higher doses.

7. _____ is a fatal symptom often associated with an overdose of barbiturates or other CNS depressants.

8. Schedule _____ is the level assigned to many benzodiazepines; Schedule _____ is the level assigned to some barbiturates.

9. _____ is a form of depression associated with reduced release of melatonin.

10. Non-REM and REM sleep are most affected by _____ drugs.

MATCHING

For questions 11 through 15, match the descriptions in column I with its drug classification in column II.

Column I

11. _____ Beginning in the early 1900s, the drug classification that has been used to control seizures, insomnia, and anxiety

12. _____ Class containing drugs that act by binding GABA, intensifying the effect, without causing respiratory depression unless taken with other CNS depressants

13. _____ Class containing older agents rarely prescribed due to safer agents, commonly prescribed for anxiety and insomnia

14. _____ Class containing antihistamines, used in OTC sleep aids that do not cause dependency

15. _____ A chemical related to tryptophan, sold OTC

Column II

a. Benzodiazepines

b. Barbiturates

c. Nonbenzodiazepines, nonbarbiturate sedatives

d. Melatonin

e. Anticholinergics

For questions 16 through 21, match the drug in column I with its class name and most appropriate use in column II.

Column I

16. _____ Secobarbital (Seconal)

17. _____ Chlordiazepoxide (Librium)

18. _____ Zolpidem (Ambien)

19. _____ Prazepam (Centrax)

20. _____ Amobarbital (Amytal)

21. _____ Triazolam (Halcion)

Column II

a. Benzodiazepine for anxiety and panic

b. Benzodiazepine for short-term relief of insomnia

c. Barbiturate for short-term relief of insomnia

d. Barbiturate for short-term sedation

e. Nonbarbiturate CNS depressant for short-term relief of insomnia

MULTIPLE CHOICE

22. What term describes episodes of immediate and intense apprehension, fearfulness, or terror?

   a. Anxiety

   b. Panic

   c. Phobia

   d. Posttraumatic stress

23. What drugs are meant to address anxiety on a more limited basis?

   a. Anxiolytics

   b. Sedatives

   c. Mood disorder drugs

   d. Antidepressants

24. Benzodiazepines have several uses. Which would be an inappropriate use?

    a. Long-term administration to treat phobias, OCD, and PTSD

    b. When anxiety interferes with daily activities of living

    c. Short-term treatment of generalized anxiety disorder

    d. Short-term treatment of insomnia caused by anxiety

25. Which of the following terms may be used to describe benzodiazepines?

    a. Sedative

    b. Hypnotic

    c. Tranquilizer

    d. All of the above

26. What was one of the first drugs used for anxiety treatment?

    a. Alprazolam (Xanax)

    b. Clonazepam (Klonopin)

    c. Chlordiazepoxide (Librium)

    d. Clorazepate (Tranxene)

27. CNS depressants include which of the following drug classes?

    a. Benzodiazepines

    b. Barbiturates

    c. Nonbarbiturates, nonbenzodiazepine sedatives

    d. All of the above

28. Which statement is true about reestablishing a healthful sleep regimen?

    a. Drinking alcohol close to bedtime helps one to sleep.

    b. Eating a moderate meal close to bedtime helps one to sleep.

    c. Supplements are often recommended for insomnia.

    d. Sedatives and hypnotics may be useful for insomnia if taken long term.

29. Which of the following best describes rebound insomnia?

    a. A time during which insomnia and symptoms of anxiety may worsen

    b. A worsening of insomnia due to drug dependency

    c. More common in younger patients

    d. Develops from short-term use of insomnia medication

30. Melatonin can be bought OTC for insomnia. Which patient teaching would be appropriate?

    a. Melatonin can increase ovulation in women trying to conceive.

    b. Melatonin can be taken safely during pregnancy.

    c. Melatonin can safely be given to patients who are on steroids.

    d. Melatonin is not regulated by the FDA, but sold OTC without a prescription.

31. Which of the following is true regarding sleep stages and patterns?

    a. Drugs for insomnia generally do not affect sleep stages.

    b. Patients with normal sleep patterns move from non-REM to REM sleep about every 90 minutes.

    c. REM sleep is the deepest stage of sleep.

    d. The most significant type of sleep with respect to the effect of hypnotic drugs is REM sleep.

32. Sleep deprivation has been linked to which of the following?

    a. Decreased risk of type 2 diabetes

    b. Becoming frightened, irritable, paranoid, and emotionally disturbed

    c. Less daydreaming or fantasizing throughout the day

    d. Better judgment and less impulsive thinking

33. Which of the following best describes phenobarbital?

    a. Is a short-acting barbiturate and thus more useful for brief medical procedures

    b. Stimulates liver enzymes and thus may increase its own metabolism with repeated dosing

    c. Is mainly limited in drug therapy for induction of sleep

    d. Doses not affect levels of folate (B_9) or vitamin D in the body

34. Benzodiazepines must be given with caution when given parenterally due to what risk?

    a. Seizures

    b. CNS excitation

    c. Respiratory depression

    d. Dependence

35. Which of the following best describes buspirone (BuSpar)?

    a. Is a benzodiazepine

    b. May act by binding to brain dopamine and serotonin receptors

    c. Is used for short-term treatment of insomnia

    d. All of the above

MAKING CONNECTIONS

36. A patient is experiencing extreme anxiety in a dental chair due to an impending tooth extraction. Which route should the dentist use to give the most rapid onset of action?

    a. Oral

    b. IV

    c. IM

    d. Rectal

37. Scopolamine (Transderm-Scop) is an anticholinergic agent. Which of the following would *least* likely be a side effect of this drug?

   a. Dry mouth

   b. Bradycardia

   c. Tachycardia

   d. Urinary retention

38. Which of the following drug delivery methods is *not* a parenteral method of drug delivery, it avoids the first-pass effect in the liver?

   a. Oral

   b. Intrathecal

   c. Intramuscular

   d. Sublingual

39. One reason the first-pass effect is so important is that drugs absorbed at the level of the digestive tract do which of the following?

   a. Are circulated directly back to the heart

   b. Are distributed to the rest of the body and target organs

   c. Have ultimately more bioavailability than they would if absorbed at a different location

   d. Are routed through the hepatic portal circulation

40. Younger and elder patients metabolize drugs _____ than middle-age patients

   a. More slowly

   b. More rapidly

   c. At the same rate

CALCULATIONS

41. A physician orders lorazepam 1.5 mg IV bolus. The pharmacy supplies 0.001 g/ml of lorazepam. The nurse

   should administer _____ ml IV bolus as ordered.

42. The physician orders diazepam 1 mg solution PO. The oral solution is 5 mg/ml. The nurse should administer

   _____ ml / dose.

CASE STUDY APPLICATIONS

43. Mr. L is a 38-year-old patient who is to have a short surgical procedure during which he will be given Versed IV. The nurse knows that Versed is a short-acting benzodiazepine.

   a. What does the nurse need to assess prior to giving Versed?

   b. What interventions would the nurse use to maintain the patient's safety during the procedure?

   c. What would the nurse use to evaluate the effectiveness of these interventions?

44. Mrs. D has not slept in weeks. She is troubled about a new job and feels that if she can just get through a couple more weeks, things might start to become a little easier. One thing that would definitely help Mrs. D is a good night's sleep.

   a. What nursing diagnosis would you identify for this patient?

   b. What nursing interventions would be used to assist this patient?

   c. What would the nurse teach the patient regarding pharmacologic interventions available?

CHAPTER 15

DRUGS FOR SEIZURES

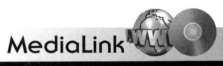

MediaLink

www.prenhall.com/adams

CD-ROM
Animation:
  Mechanism in Action: Diazepam (Valium)
Audio Glossary
NCLEX Review

Companion Website
NCLEX Review
Dosage Calculations
Care Plans
Expanded Key Concepts

OBJECTIVES

To view the objectives, please refer to the textbook, student CD-Rom, and the Companion Website at *www.prenhall.com/adams*.

FILL IN THE BLANK

From the textbook, find the correct word(s) to complete the statement(s).

1. Seizures can result from _____ situations or occur on a _____ basis as with epilepsy.

2. Five possible causes of seizures include _____ , _____ , _____ , _____ , and _____ .

3. Because antiseizure drugs are mostly pregnancy category D, patients should use _____ or other contraceptive measures.

4. Antiseizure drugs may cause _____ deficiency which can cause neural tube defects in a fetus.

5. Patients who have seizures may have a lower tolerance to environmental triggers such as _____ deprivation and exposure to _____ or _____ lights.

6. _____ seizures occur in 0.5% of _____-month-old to _____ year-old children during an illness, and last 1 to 2 minutes. Prevention is best carried out by controlling _____.

7. Of the major antiseizure medications, _____ is a drug of choice for a broader range of seizure types.

8. _____ seizures occur only on one side of the brain and continue for a short distance before they stop; _____ seizures may travel throughout the brain.

9. Of the most popular antiseizure medications, the drug of choice for absence seizures is _____.

10. Two popular medications used to treat status epilepticus are _____ and _____.

11. _____ is an emergency type of generalized tonic-clonic seizure that is prolonged and usually affects _____, causing hypoxia.

12. If not treated, status epilepticus can cause _____ damage or death.

13. Treatment of status epilepticus includes maintenance of the _____ and IV antiseizure medications.

14. Abrupt discontinuation of antiseizure medications could cause _____.

15. The goal of antiseizure medications is to prevent _____ or repeated firing and therefore to _____ neuronal activity.

16. Once seizures are controlled, drug therapy continues for some time. After _____ years, the medications may be withdrawn slowly, one at a time, over several _____.

MATCHING

For questions 17 through 23, match the signs and symptoms in column I with its type of seizure in column II.

Column I

17. _____ In adults, this seizure may be preceded by an aura. Muscles then become tense, and a rhythmic jerking motion develops.

18. _____ This seizure is marked by major muscle groups contracting quickly, making a jerking motion. Patients appear unsteady and clumsy and may fall from a sitting position or drop whatever they are holding.

19. _____ This seizure usually starts with a blank stare. Patients may become disoriented and not pay attention to verbal commands or act as if they have a psychiatric illness. After the seizure, patients do not remember what happened.

20. _____ Patients may feel for a brief moment that their precise location is vague and out of sorts. Often patients will hear and see things that are not there or may smell or taste things and have an upset stomach. Parts of the body such as the arms, legs, or face may start twitching. Symptoms are often not dramatic and may occur without loss of consciousness.

Column II

a. Simple partial seizure

b. Complex partial seizure (psychomotor or temporal lobe seizure)

c. Absence seizure (petit mal seizure)

d. Atonic seizure (drop attack)

e. Myoclonic seizure

f. Generalized tonic-clonic seizure (grand mal seizure)

g. Status epilepticus

21. _____ This type of seizure occurs most often in children. Patients develop a blank stare without having twitching facial or body movements. This seizure lasts for only a few seconds. Patients then quickly recover and engage in normal activities.

22. _____ This is a medical emergency brought on by repeated seizures and convulsions. Steps must be taken to ensure that the airway remains open.

23. _____ Patients often stumble or fall for no apparent reason. Episodes are very short, lasting only a matter of seconds. After the seizure, patients return to normal activities without difficulty.

For questions 24 through 29, match the drug in column I with its pharmacologic category in column II.

Column I	**Column II**
24. _____ Phenobarbital (Luminal)	a. Drugs acting through a GABA receptor
25. _____ Clonazepam (Klonopin)	b. Drugs delaying an influx of sodium across neuronal membranes
26. _____ Phenytoin (Dilantin)	
27. _____ Gabapentin (Neurontin)	c. Drugs delaying an influx of calcium across neuronal membranes
28. _____ Carbamazepine (Tegretol)	
29. _____ Ethosuximide (Zarontin)	

MULTIPLE CHOICE

30. What common concern occurs with phenobarbital (Luminal)?

    a. Irregular heart beat

    b. Blood cell reactions

    c. Hypotension

    d. Vitamin D and folate deficiency

31. What is the main advantage of using carbamazepine (Tegretol) for partial seizures?

    a. Category C status

    b. Dual use for the treatment of trigeminal neuralgia

    c. Ability to cause less drowsiness

    d. Dual use for the treatment of manic-depressive disorder

32. Which one of the following is the newest hydantoin-like drug?

    a. Phenytoin (Dilantin)

    b. Zonisamide (Zonegran)

    c. Carbamazepine (Tegretol)

    d. Valproic acid (Depakene)

33. Which of the following medications is used to treat Lennox-Gastaut syndrome?

    a. Fosphenytoin (Cerebyx)

    b. Felbamate (Felbatol)

    c. Lamotrigine (Lamictal)

    d. Methsuximide (Celontin)

34. Which antiseizure medication might produce psychotic behavior symptoms?

    a. Ethosuximide (Zarontin)

    b. Amobarbital (Amytal)

    c. Lorazepam (Ativan)

    d. Gabapentin (Neurontin)

35. Which is the most potent benzodiazepine used for the treatment of convulsions?

    a. Clonazepam (Klonopin)

    b. Clorazepate (Tranxene)

    c. Diazepam (Valium)

    d. Lorazepam (Ativan)

36. Which of the following medications is converted to phenytoin in the body?

    a. Fosphenytoin (Cerebyx)

    b. Felbamate (Felbatol)

    c. Divalproex (Depakote)

    d. Lamotrigine (Lamictal)

37. What is the major concern in making antiseizure therapy successful?

    a. Avoiding kidney and liver toxicity

    b. Making sure the patient complies with medication

    c. Maintaining proper drug levels in the bloodstream

    d. All of the above

38. Why should women of childbearing age be counseled regarding antiseizure medications?

    a. They are teratogenic.

    b. They interfere with oral contraceptives.

    c. They produce folic acid deficiency.

    d. All of the above.

39. Patients taking barbiturates for seizures must be monitored for respiratory depression in the presence of which of the following?

    a. Oral administration

    b. Nonopiate analgesics

    c. Chronic respiratory dysfunction

    d. All of the above

40. A patient is admitted with an overdose of Valium. Which of the following drugs would the nurse need to have on hand?

    a. Diphenhydramine (Benadryl)

    b. Flumazenil (Romazicon)

    c. Epinephrine

    d. Atropine

41. The nurse should teach the patient taking benzodiazepines that the drug can do which of the following?

    a. Cause sedation when first started

    b. Be safely stopped abruptly

    c. Increase the amount of digoxin needed

    d. Be potentiated by smoking, nicotine patches, or chewing tobacco

42. A patient taking phenytoin (Dilantin) chronically for seizures should be encouraged to maintain good oral hygiene and visit the dentist every 6 months. Phenytoin does which of the following in patients?

    a. Causes cavities

    b. Causes gingival hyperplasia

    c. Causes mouth cancers

    d. Builds up tartar on the teeth

MAKING CONNECTIONS

43. Although phenobarbital is an antiseizure medicine, it is also classified as which of the following?

    a. Benzodiazepine

    b. Category I drug

    c. Sympathomimetic

    d. Sedative-hypnotic

44. Which term describes a craving of a patient to continue drug use despite its negative effects?

    a. Tolerance

    b. Physical dependence

    c. Psychologic dependence

    d. Resistance

45. When are seizures in a patient who is undergoing alcohol withdrawal most likely to occur?

    a. Immediately after the patient has stopped drinking

    b. 1 to 3 days after the patient has stopped drinking

    c. 5 to 7 days after the patient has stopped drinking

    d. During an episode of delirium tremens (DTs)

46. Which of the following drugs is not used to treat convulsions?

    a. Buspirone (BuSpar)

    b. Phenobarbital (Luminal)

    c. Gabapentin (Neurontin)

    d. Carbamazepine (Tegretol)

47. What is the most important reason why benzodiazepines are not used for chronic seizure control?

    a. Tendency for the patient to develop tolerance to the drug

    b. Psychologic addiction

    c. Respiratory depression that occurs in chronic use

    d. No antidote exists

CALCULATIONS

48. The physician orders phenobarbital elixir 60 mg PO bid. The pharmacy fills the prescription with phenobarbital elixir 20 mg/5 ml. The patient's care provider should be instructed to administer _____ ml per dose.

49. The physician orders felbamate (Felbatol) 1200 mg per day in four divided doses. The nurse would give _____ mg per dose?

CASE STUDY APPLICATIONS

50. A nurse is preparing for a patient who is coming to the ER with status epilepticus. The physician has ordered Dilantin by IV drip as soon as the patient arrives.

    a. What evidence (assessment data) would support a nursing diagnosis of "risk for injury?"

    b. What interventions would provide safety for the patient during Dilantin administration?

51. A male patient has been placed on Dilantin for newly diagnosed epilepsy. He has generalized tonic-clonic seizures. He has asked how long it will take to manage his seizures and what side effects can occur. He also wants to know what foods or drugs to avoid while on this medication.

    a. Which nursing diagnosis would be top priority for this patient?

    b. What interventions would be helpful for this diagnosis?

CHAPTER 16

DRUGS FOR EMOTIONAL AND MOOD DISORDERS

OBJECTIVES

To view the objectives, please refer to the textbook, student CD-ROM, and the Companion Website at *www.prenhall.com/adams*.

FILL IN THE BLANK

From the textbook, find the correct word(s) to complete the statement(s).

1. Another name for mood disorders is _____ disorders.

2. The two major types of mood disorders are _____ and
   _____.

3. The three major classes of antidepressants are _____,
   _____ and _____.

4. _____ are drugs of choice for simple depression.

5. _____ produce fewer cardiovascular side effects, and therefore are less dangerous than the MAOIs.

6. Patients taking _____ for bipolar disorder should be placed on a low-sodium diet to increase its effectiveness.

7. The inability to focus or pay attention is one of the main symptoms of _____.

8. _____ are the class of drugs most widely prescribed for ADHD.

9. _____ disorder is depression associated with reduced release of melatonin during winter months.

10. Drugs for bipolar disorders are called _____ because they have the ability to modulate extreme
    shifts in emotions between _____ and _____.

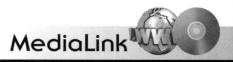

MediaLink

www.prenhall.com/adams

CD-ROM
Animations:
   Mechanism in Action: Fluoxetine (Prozac)
   Mechanism in Action: Methylphenidate
   (Ritalin)
Audio Glossary
NCLEX Review

Companion Website
NCLEX Review
Dosage Calculations
Case Study
Expanded Key Concepts

MATCHING

For questions 11 through 22, match the drug in column I with its primary indication or class in column II.

Column I	Column II
11. _____ Lithium carbonate (Eskalith)	a. ADD/CNS stimulant
12. _____ Venlafaxine (Effexor)	b. Depression/tricyclic type
13. _____ Paroxetine (Paxil)	c. Depression/MAOI
14. _____ Amitriptyline hydrochloride (Elavil)	d. Depression/SSRI
15. _____ Phenelzine sulfate (Nardil)	e. Depression/atypical or other
16. _____ Methylphenidate hydrochloride (Ritalin)	f. Bipolar disorder
17. _____ Pemoline (Cylert)	
18. _____ Tranylcypromine sulfate (Parnate)	
19. _____ Nortriptyline hydrochloride (Aventyl, Pamelor)	
20. _____ Bupropion hydrochloride (Wellbutrin)	
21. _____ Fluoxetine hydrochloride (Prozac)	
22. _____ Sertraline hydrochloride (Zoloft)	

For questions 23 through 27, match the definition in column I with its correct term in column II.

Column I	Column II
23. _____ Enzyme that breaks down cathecholamine neurotransmitters in the synapse	a. Amphetamines
24. _____ Accumulation of serotonin when taking two drugs that reduce serotonin uptake	b. Bipolar disorder
25. _____ Condition exhibiting signs of both clinical depression and mania	c. Monoamine oxidase
26. _____ The class of drug that is closely related to methylphenidate	d. Tyramine
27. _____ Chemical found in medications that cannot be ingested by patients on MAOIs due to high risk of severe hypertension	e. Serotonin syndrome

MULTIPLE CHOICE

28. What is the most common age range for the diagnosis of attention-deficit disorder (ADD)?

    a. 0 to 3 years

    b. 3 to 7 years

    c. 10 to 13 years

    d. 15 to 18 years

29. Which medication has *not* been useful in stabilizing emotions in mood disorders such as bipolar disorder?

    a. Lithium (Eskalith)

    b. Carbamazepine (Tegretol)

    c. Valproic acid (Depakene)

    d. Pemoline (Cylert)

30. Lithium is used with other medications during phases of bipolar disorder. The nurse knows that which of these medications would *not* be used with lithium?

    a. Tricyclic antidepressants

    b. Benzodiazepines

    c. SSRI antidepressants

    d. Diuretics

31. Which of the following is an advantage of using Scattera instead of a scheduled CNS stimulant?

    a. Scattera improves ability to focus and decreases hyperactivity.

    b. Scattera has shown more efficacy than Ritalin.

    c. Scattera has fewer CNS side effects than Ritalin.

    d. Scattera is not as addictive as Ritalin.

32. A patient is sent home after being given fluoxetine (Prozac) for depression. The nurse should instruct the patient to do which of the following?

    a. Call back if there is no improvement in 24 hours.

    b. Call back if any nausea, drowsiness, or dizziness occurs.

    c. Start the Prozac before stopping the patient's present MAOI.

    d. Expect to see improvement in mood, appetite, and energy within 1 to 3 weeks.

33. Methylphenidate (Ritalin) produces its effects by activating what portion of the brain?

    a. Cerebellum

    b. Hypothalamus

    c. Pituitary

    d. Reticular activating system

34. When sending a patient home on imipramine (Tofranil), which of the following is important for the nurse to teach patients?

    a. St. John's wort may be used concurrently with no anticipated interaction.

    b. Photosensitivy is not a problem with Tofranil.

    c. This drug should not be stopped abruptly.

    d. Use of this drug with other CNS depressants is permitted.

35. Which of the following is *not* a common symptom of clinical depression?

    a. Lack of energy

    b. Sleep disturbances

c. Hallucinations

d. Feelings of despair or guilt

36. In assessing a patient, the nurse should know that rapid shifts in emotions from profound depression to euphoria and hyperactivity are characteristic of which of the following?

a. Psychosis

b. Bipolar disorder

c. Schizophrenia

d. ADD

37. Which of the following would *least* likely be used to treat clinical depression?

a. Monoamine oxidase inhibitors

b. Tricyclic antidepressants

c. Selective serotonin reuptake inhibitors

d. Phenothiazines

38. How does phenelzine (Nardil) produce its therapeutic effects?

a. Inhibits the reuptake of norepinephrine into presynaptic nerve terminals

b. Irreversibly inhibits monoamine oxidase (MAO) and intensifies the effects of norepinephrine in the synapse

c. Selectively inhibits the reuptake of serotonin into presynaptic nerve terminals

d. Interferes with the binding of dopamine to receptors located in the limbic system

39. How do tricyclic antidepressants produce their therapeutic effects?

a. Inhibit the reuptake of both serotonin and norepinephrine into presynaptic nerve terminals

b. Irreversibly inhibit monoamine oxidase (MAO) and intensify the effects of norepinephrine in the synapse

c. Selectively inhibit the reuptake of serotonin into presynaptic nerve terminals

d. Interfere with the binding of dopamine to receptors located in the limbic system

40. How does fluoxetine (Prozac) produce its therapeutic effects?

a. Inhibit the reuptake of both serotonin and norepinephrine into presynaptic nerve terminals

b. Irreversibly inhibits monoamine oxidase (MAO) and intensifies the effects of norepinephrine in the synapse

c. Selectively inhibits the reuptake of serotonin into presynaptic nerve terminals

d. Interferes with the binding of dopamine to receptors located in the limbic system

41. Why are the selective serotonin reuptake inhibitors (SSRIs) generally preferred over other classes of antidepressants?

a. More efficacious

b. Produce fewer sympathomimetic and anticholinergic side effects

c. Do not produce sexual dysfunction

d. Cause more extrapyramidal effects

42. The nurse should teach patients taking fluoxetine to avoid foods high in which amino acid, because it is a chemical precursor for serotonin synthesis?

    a. Histidine

    b. Tyramine

    c. Lysine

    d. Tryptophan

MAKING CONNECTIONS

43. Typical oral doses are 1 mg for risperidone and 50 mg for clozapine. Which of the following may you correctly conclude from this information?

    a. Risperidone is more efficacious.

    b. Clozapine is more efficacious.

    c. Risperidone is more potent.

    d. Clozapine is more potent.

44. Thorazine is available by both IM and oral routes. Which would be expected to have a faster onset of action?

    a. IM

    b. Oral

45. In assessing a new patient, the nurse should know that panic attacks, phobias, and obsessive-compulsive disorders are usually treated with which of the following?

    a. Antipsychotic drugs

    b. Antianxiety drugs

    c. Drugs for bipolar disorder

    d. Antidepressants

46. "Speedball" is the street name for a drug combination containing methylphenidate (Ritalin) and which of the following?

    a. Heroin

    b. Marijuana

    c. LSD

    d. Cocaine

47. Methylphenidate is a Schedule II drug. What does this mean?

    a. It may adversely affect the fetus.

    b. It has no therapeutic use.

    c. It has a low abuse potential.

    d. It has a high potential for physical and psychological dependence.

CALCULATIONS

48. The physician orders lithium carbonate 1.2 g PO qd in four divided doses. The pharmacy supplies 300 mg lithium carbonate capsules. The nurse should instruct the patient to take _____ capsule per dose.

49. The physician orders fluoxetine 45 mg PO qd. The pharmacy fills the prescription with fluoxetine oral solution .of 20 mg/5 ml. The patient should be instructed to take _____ ml per day.

CASE STUDY APPLICATIONS

50. A patient who has bipolar disorder has been started on lithium. He is also on paroxetine (Paxil), digoxin (Lanoxin), furosemide (Lasix), and potassium supplements for depression, hypertension, and CHF. He has also been on a low-sodium diet.

    a. During the first 3 weeks on lithium, what would the nurse identify as the priority nursing diagnosis?

    b. What assessments would the nurse make in identifying this diagnosis?

    c. What is the patient goal for the first 3 weeks of therapy?

51. A patient, Mrs. C, has been started on sertraline (Zoloft) for depression. Upon being admitted, she has been assessed as having episodes of crying, feelings of guilt, insomnia, and suicidal ideation. The nurse needs to monitor the patient for effectiveness, side effects, and potential problems. Discuss what goals might be assigned the patient and how those goals could be evaluated.

CHAPTER 17

DRUGS FOR PSYCHOSES

OBJECTIVES

To view the objectives, please refer to the textbook, student CD-ROM, and the Companion Website at *www.prenhall.com/adams*.

FILL IN THE BLANK

From the textbook, find the correct word(s) to complete the statement(s).

1. The most common type of psychosis is _____.

2. Psychoses may be classified as _____ or

   _____.

3. Chronic psychoses develops over _____, whereas acute psychoses develops in _____.

4. Atypical antipsychotic drugs are effective for both _____ or _____ symptoms of psychosis.

5. The majority of psychoses have no known _____. The six identifiable causes are _____,

   _____, _____, _____, _____, or _____.

6. Positive symptoms include _____, _____, _____, and _____.

7. Negative symptoms include a lack of _____, _____, _____, and _____.

8. Proper diagnosis of positive and negative symptoms is important for selection of the appropriate

   _____ drugs.

9. Symptoms of schizophrenia are thought to be associated with the _____ receptors in the basal nuclei.

10. Medications that block 65% of D2 receptors will reduce symptoms of _____. Blocking more

    than 80% will likely cause _____ symptoms.

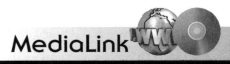

MediaLink

www.prenhall.com/adams

CD-ROM
Animation: Extrapyramidal Signs (EPS)
Audio Glossary
NCLEX Review

Companion Website
NCLEX Review
Dosage Calculations
Case Study
Care Plans
Expanded Key Concepts

MATCHING

For questions 11 through 20, match the drug in column I with its primary indication or class in column II.

Column I	Column II
11. _____ Haloperidol (Haldol)	a. Psychosis/phenothiazine
12. _____ Thioridazine (Mellaril)	b. Psychosis/nonphenothiazine
13. _____ Chlorpromazine (Thorazine)	c. Psychosis/atypical
14. _____ Prochlorperazine (Compazine)	d. Dopamine system stabilizers
15. _____ Olanzapine (Zyprexa)	
16. _____ Loxapine (Loxitane)	
17. _____ Clozapine (Clozaril)	
18. _____ Aripiprazole (Abilify)	
19. _____ Thiothixene (Navane)	
20. _____ Risperidone (Risperdal)	

For questions 21 through 29, match the characteristics in column I with their terms and conditions in column II.

Column I	Column II
21. _____ A condition in which the patient exhibits symptoms of both schizophrenia and mood disorders	a. Paranoid
22. _____ Firm ideas and beliefs not founded in reality	b. Delusions
23. _____ Symptoms that are added to normal behavior	c. Hallucinations
24. _____ A term meaning "antipsychotic medications"	d. Positive symptoms
25. _____ An extreme suspicion that one is being followed, or that others are trying to harm oneself	e. Negative symptoms
26. _____ Symptoms that subtract from a normal behavior	f. Schizoaffective disorders
27. _____ Seeing, hearing, or feeling something that is not there	g. Neuroleptic
28. _____ A class of drug that might be used to decrease extrapyramidal effects	h. Anticholinergics
29. _____ A movement disorder brought on by medication effects	i. Extrapyramidal effects

MULTIPLE CHOICE

30. Which class of drugs tends to produce severe side effects such as muscle twitching, compulsive motor activity, and a Parkinson-like syndrome?

    a. Barbiturates

    b. Phenothiazines

    c. Benzodiazepines

    d. Serotonin reuptake inhibitors

31. Delusions, hallucinations, disordered communication, and difficulty relating to others are symptoms closely associated with which of the following?

    a. Clinical depression

    b. Bipolar disorder

    c. Schizophrenia

    d. ADD

32. Which term/phrase best describes extrapyramidal side effects?

    a. Paranoid delusions

    b. Profound depression

    c. Seizures

    d. Distorted body movements and muscle spasms

33. Like many antipsychotics, chlorpromazine (Thorazine) usually takes how long before its therapeutic effect is achieved?

    a. 2 to 3 days

    b. 2 to 3 weeks

    c. 7 to 8 weeks

    d. More than 6 months

34. Many of the major effects of chlorpromazine (Thorazine) can be attributed to which of the following?

    a. Inhibiting the reuptake of both serotonin and norepinephrine into presynaptic nerve terminals

    b. Irreversibly inhibiting monoamine oxidase (MAO) and intensifying the effects of norepinephrine in the synapse

    c. Selectively inhibiting the reuptake of serotonin into presynaptic nerve terminals

    d. Interfering with the binding of dopamine to receptors located throughout the brain

35. Why are atypical antipsychotics sometimes preferred over phenothiazines?

    a. They produce no major adverse effects.

    b. They can treat both positive and negative symptoms of psychosis.

    c. They are much more efficacious.

    d. They can improve symptoms within a few days of initial administration.

36. Nonphenothiazine agents differ from phenothiazine agents in what way?

   a. Nonphenothiazines do not produce as many anticholinergic side effects as phenothiazines.

   b. Nonphenothiazines cause less sedation and fewer anticholinergic side effects than phenothiazines.

   c. Phenothiazines do not produce as many side effects as nonphenothiazines.

   d. Phenothiazines cause less sedation and anticholinergic side effects than nonphenothiazines.

37. Patients on clozapine (Clozaril) must watch carefully for signs of agranulocytosis, which include which of the following?

   a. Dizziness and drowsiness

   b. Appetite increase

   c. Fever and sore throat

   d. Bruises and bleeding

38. A patient who is on a phenothiazine complains of having elevated temperature, sweating, and "not feeling well." What possible indication should the nurse assess the patient for?

   a. Agranulocytosis

   b. Neuroleptic malignant syndrome

   c. Infection that may decrease potency of the medication

   d. Dystonic reaction

39. For a patient who has problems with daily compliance, a drug is available that lasts for 3 weeks. Which drug would be a good choice for this patient?

   a. Haloperidol (Haldol LA)

   b. Olanzapine (Zyprexa)

   c. Chlorpromazine (Thorazine)

   d. Clozapine (Clozaril)

MAKING CONNECTIONS

40. A patient has been prescribed an antipsychotic drug that has a high degree of anticholinergic side effects. Anticholinergic effects include which of the following?

   a. Nervousness and tremors

   b. Restlessness and constant movement of legs

   c. Drying of mouth, sedation, and urinary retention

   d. Headaches, skin rashes, and hallucinations

41. The atypical antipsychotics bind to serotonergic and cholinergic sites throughout the brain. The nurse understands that this would affect which neurotransmitters?

   a. Acetylcholine and serotonin

   b. Serotonin and dopamine

   c. Serotonin and norepinephrine

   d. Acetylcholine and norepinephrine

42. Benzodiazepines are often given with antipsychotic drugs. Which benzodiazepine side effects would create a problem when given with this class of antipsychotic medications?

    a. Drowsiness and dry mouth

    b. Lowered seizure threshold

    c. Hypotension and respiratory depression

    d. Bone marrow depression

43. Patients on herbal supplements must be warned about interactions with other prescribed medications. What herbal preparations are sometimes taken to treat mental illness?

    a. Tryptophan

    b. St. John's wart

    c. Kava

    d. All of the above

44. Schizoaffective disorder is treated with antipsychotic medications and may require antidepressants. Which of the following medications is an antidepressant?

    a. Diazepam (Valium)

    b. Phenytoin (Dilantin)

    c. Chlorpromazine (Thorazine)

    d. Paroxetine (Paxil)

CALCULATIONS

45. The physician orders fluphenazine 15 mg SC. The pharmacy supplies fluphenazine 25 mg/ml. The nurse would administer _____ ml SC.

46. A patient has an order for Seroquel 200 mg/day in divided dosages bid. Seroquel comes in 50 mg tablets. How many tablets would the nurse give per dose _____?

CASE STUDY APPLICATIONS

47. Mrs. S has been taking Thorazine for about a year. She has been having problems with orthostatic hypotension and akathisia, and has needed to take Cogentin to avoid dystonic reactions. The physician has decided to change her to Clozaril. The patient asks the nurse about the advantages and disadvantages of the new drug. The nurse has chosen knowledge deficit as the nursing diagnosis for this patient.

    a. What interventions would be used for this diagnosis?

    b. How would the nurse evaluate the outcome of the interventions?

48. Ms. G has recently been diagnosed with schizophrenia. She has been placed on Haldol while hospitalized, and has had hallucinations and delusions. What assessments would the nurse need to complete during the first 3 weeks that the patient is on this medication?

CHAPTER 18

DRUGS FOR DEGENERATIVE DISEASES OF THE NERVOUS SYSTEM

OBJECTIVES

To view the objectives, please refer to the textbook, student CD-ROM, and the Companion Website at *www.prenhall.com/adams*.

FILL IN THE BLANK

From the textbook, find the correct word(s) to complete the statement(s).

1. A patient with Parkinson's disease may experience difficulty urinating and performing sexually, which are signs of disturbances of the _____ nervous system.

2. Drug therapy of Parkinson's disease focuses on restoring dopamine function and also blocking the effect of _____ within the same area of the brain.

3. _____ is a degenerative disorder characterized by progressive memory loss, confusion, and inability to think or communicate effectively.

4. The most common causes of dementia are _____ and _____.

5. Alzheimer's patients experience a dramatic loss of their ability to perform tasks that require _____ as a neurotransmitter.

6. Parkinson's disease could be related to a _____ link since many patients have a family history of the disorder.

7. Extensive treatment with certain _____ medications may induce Parkinson-like syndrome or _____ symptoms.

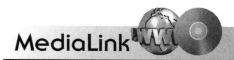

8. Side effects of drugs used to treat parkinsonism include _____ and _____. Signs of toxicity would include _____ and _____.

9. When treating Alzheimer's disease, the goal of pharmacotherapy is to improve the function in three domains: _____, _____, and _____.

10. _____ can only be used in the early stages of Alzheimer's because they are only effective in the presence of _____ neurons.

MATCHING

For questions 11 through 20, match the drug in column I with its primary classification in column II.

Column I	Column II
11. _____ Biperiden hydrochloride (Akineton)	a. Dopaminergic drug
12. _____ Levodopa (L-Dopa, Larodopa)	b. Cholinergic blocking drug
13. _____ Tacrine (Cognex)	c. Cholinergic drug (AchE inhibitor)
14. _____ Pergolide (Permax)	
15. _____ Benztropine (Cogentin)	
16. _____ Donepezil (Aricept)	
17. _____ Bromocriptine (Parlodel)	
18. _____ Tolcapone (Tasmar)	
19. _____ Procyclidine (Kemadrin)	
20. _____ Galantamine (Reminyl)	

For questions 21 through 29, match the characteristics in column I with their drugs in column II.

Column I	Column II
21. _____ Decreases effect of dopaminergics	a. Levodopa
22. _____ Antioxidant possibly useful in Alzheimer's disease	b. Sinemet
23. _____ Approved in Europe for dementia but not yet in the United States; can react with anticoagulants	c. Selegiline
24. _____ Antiviral that releases dopamine from its nerve terminals	d. Bromocriptine
25. _____ Acetylcholinesterase inhibitor used for Alzheimer's associated with hepatotoxicity	e. Amantadine
26. _____ Drug of choice for Parkinsonism	f. Tacrine
27. _____ Inhibits enzymes that destroy levodopa or dopamine	g. Ginkgo biloba
28. _____ Dopamine agonist that activates the dopamine receptors	h. Donepezil
29. _____ Carbidopa that is added to levodopa to make more levodopa available to enter the CNS	i. Pyridoxine

MULTIPLE CHOICE

30. Parkinson's disease is a degenerative disorder of the nervous system caused by the death of neurons that produce which of the following?

    a. Dopamine

    b. Norepinephrine

    c. Acetylcholine

    d. Serotonin

31. A patient is admitted with a new diagnosis of Parkinson's disease. If he is in the early stages, what would usually *not* be seen on assessment?

    a. Tremor

    b. Muscle rigidity and weakness

    c. Bradykinesia

    d. Dementia

32. What is the relationship between acetylcholine and dopamine in the area of the brain that affects balance, posture, and involuntary muscle movement?

    a. Both dopamine and acetylcholine stimulate this region.

    b. Both dopamine and acetylcholine inhibit this region.

    c. Dopamine stimulates and acetylcholine inhibits this region.

    d. Dopamine inhibits and acetylcholine stimulates this region.

33. What class of drugs may induce artificial parkinsonism by interfering with the same neural pathway and functions modified by a lack of dopamine?

    a. Phenothiazines

    b. Tricyclic antidepressants

    c. MAO inhibitors

    d. Benzodiazepines

34. A patient develops EPS after taking phenothiazines. The nurse would expect an order for which medication to counteract the EPS?

    a. Diphenhydramine (Benadryl)

    b. Procyclidine (Kemadrin)

    c. Levodopa (Larodopa)

    d. Tacrine (Cognex)

35. Which drug has been prescribed more extensively than any other drug for patients with Parkinson's disease?

    a. Carbidopa (Lodosyn)

    b. Benztropine (Cogentin)

    c. Levodopa (Larodopa)

    d. Tacrine (Cognex)

36. A patient is started on levodopa for Parkinson's disease. What type of side effects would be expected?

    a. Sleep disorders such as insomnia

    b. Sedation

    c. Involuntary muscle movements

    d. Seizures

37. If a patient is unable to tolerate dopaminergic medications, which class of drugs would likely be prescribed?

    a. Cholinergic drugs

    b. Anticholinergic drugs

    c. Antipsychotic drugs

    d. Selective serotonin reuptake inhibitors (SSRIs)

38. What normally causes vascular dementia?

    a. Multiple strokes

    b. Multiple heart attacks

    c. Too little blood flow to the brain

    d. Lack of sufficient neurotransmitters in certain areas of the brain

39. Amyloid plaques and neurofibrillary tangles within the brain are diagnostic signs of which of the following?

    a. Parkinson's disease

    b. Tardive dyskinesia

    c. Vascular dementia

    d. Alzheimer's disease

40. Acetylcholine inhibitors enhance the action of what chemical in the brain?

    a. Dopamine

    b. Norepinephrine

    c. Acetylcholine

    d. Serotonin

41. Drugs that inhibit the enzyme acetylcholinesterase (AchE) will do which of the following?

    a. Increase levels of dopamine

    b. Decrease levels of dopamine

    c. Increase levels of acetylcholine

    d. Decrease levels of acetylcholine

42. When a patient takes phenothiazines for an extended time, what conditions would the nurse expect to see?

    a. Parkinsonism

    b. Hypertensive crisis

    c. Decreased muscle rigidity

    d. Bruising and bleeding from the gums

MAKING CONNECTIONS

43. An anticholinergic drug is one that blocks the effects of which of the following?

    a. Epinephrine

    b. Norepinephrine

    c. Acetylcholine

    d. Serotonin

44. Succinimides, barbiturates, and benzodiazepines are used to treat what disorder?

    a. Anxiety

    b. Seizures

    c. Sleep disorders

    d. Mood disorders

45. Tacrine is highly metabolized by the liver. During the process of metabolism, what happens to the medication?

    a. It is absorbed into the bloodstream.

    b. It is excreted from the body.

    c. It is added to plasma proteins.

    d. It is made more or less active.

46. Which type of drug is given to discourage tardive dyskinesias in patients being treated for psychosis?

    a. Cholinergic

    b. Anticholinergics

    c. Dopaminergics

    d. Selective serotonin uptake inhibitors

47. Antipsychotic medications have actions that decrease which of the following in the brain?

    a. Dopamine

    b. Acetylcholine

    c. Norepinephrine

    d. Acetylcholinesterase

CALCULATIONS

48. A patient has an order for tolcapone (Tasmar) 100 mg tid. The drug is available in 25 mg tablets. How many tablets would the nurse give per day?

49. A patient has an order for Artane 7.5 mg per day. He is to take it tid. He should take _____ mg/dose?

CASE STUDY APPLICATIONS

50. Mr. H is a 30-year-old patient who has recently been diagnosed with early Parkinson's disease. He has been quite upset and depressed about the diagnosis and has lost interest in most of his usual activities and hobbies. His wife reports that his tremors and involuntary movements have worsened. He has been taking the following medications for 6 months: levodopa (2 g/day) and sertraline (Zoloft). He now has Cogentin added to his medications.

    a. What is the nursing diagnosis that best describes problems related to his condition and his new medication?

    b. What goal would relate to the diagnosis?

51. Mr. B has been brought to your facility by his wife. He was diagnosed last year with Alzheimer's disease. His confusion has become increasingly worse. He has been restless, agitated, and experiencing hallucinations. This past year, he has been taking moderate doses of amitriptyline (Elavil) and alprazolam (Xanax).
    The patient is now placed on donepezil (Aricept) for a trial. During the first 4 weeks of the treatment with this AchE inhibitor, monitoring for adverse reactions and effectiveness is the responsibility of the nurse.

    a. What would be the priority nursing diagnosis for this situation?

    b. What interventions would be included?

CHAPTER 19

DRUGS FOR THE CONTROL OF PAIN

OBJECTIVES

To view the objectives, please refer to the textbook, student CD-ROM, and the Companion Website at *www.prenhall.com/adams*.

FILL IN THE BLANK

From the textbook, find the correct word(s) to complete the statement(s).

1. The two main classes of pain medications are the

   _____ and _____.

2. All nonsteroidal anti-inflammatory drugs (NSAIDs) have

   _____ and _____ activity, as well as
   analgesic properties.

3. The narcotic analgesics are obtained from _____.

4. The type of headache characterized by a tightening of the muscles of the head and neck area due to stress is

   called a _____ headache.

5. A sensory cue that precedes a migraine is called a/an _____.

6. NSAIDs act by inhibiting pain mediators at the _____ level.

7. The sensation of pain is increased by _____, _____, and _____.

8. Successful choice of pain therapy is dependent on the _____ and _____ of the pain.

9. The goals of pharmacotherapy for migraine are to _____ the migraine in progress and to
   _____ migraines from occurring.

10. Two major drug classes used for migraine headaches include _____ and _____.
    Both of these are _____ agonists.

11. Triptans are 5-HT-selective, and thought to act by constricting _____.

    They are available to be administered _____, _____, or _____.

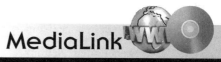

MediaLink

www.prenhall.com/adams

CD-ROM
Animation:
   Mechanism in Action: Morphine
   (Astramorph PF)
Audio Glossary
NCLEX Review

Companion Website
NCLEX Review
Dosage Calculations
Case Study
Care Plans
Expanded Key Concepts

MATCHING

For questions 12 through 23, match the drug in column I with its primary indication/class in column II.

Column I	Column II
12. _____ Naloxone (Narcan)	a. NSAID
13. _____ Meperidine (Demerol)	b. Opioid; moderate efficacy
14. _____ Celecoxib (Celebrex)	c. Opioid; high efficacy
15. _____ Oxycodone (OxyContin)	d. Opioid blocker
16. _____ Zolmitriptan (Zomig)	e. Antimigraine agent
17. _____ Nalmefene (Revex)	
18. _____ Ibuprofen (Advil, Motrin)	
19. _____ Ergotamine tartrate (Ergostat)	
20. _____ Oxymorphone (Numorphan)	
21. _____ Fenoprofen (Nalfon)	
22. _____ Propranolol (Inderal)	
23. _____ Amitriptyline (Elavil)	

For questions 24 through 29, match the description in column I with its related term in column II.

Column I	Column II
24. _____ Natural or synthetic chemicals providing pain relief	a. Nociceptor pain
25. _____ Dull, throbbing, or aching pain	b. Neuropathic pain
26. _____ Caused by injury to tissues	c. Somatic pain
27. _____ Sharp localized pain	d. Visceral pain
28. _____ Caused by injury to nerves	e. Opiates
29. _____ Natural chemicals that relieve pain	f. Opioids

MULTIPLE CHOICE

30. Painful disorders having a strong inflammatory component, such as arthritis, are treated most effectively with which of the following?

    a. NSAIDs

    b. Acetaminophen (Tylenol)

    c. Opioids

    d. Herbal supplements

31. When asked why NSAIDs are better than acetaminophen for arthritis, the healthcare provider responds, "Compared to aspirin, acetaminophen has _____."

    a. Less analgesic activity

    b. No antipyretic activity

   c. No anti-inflammatory activity

   d. The same effect on blood coagulation

32. Which of the following would be used to treat mild to moderate pain due to inflammation?

   a. Oxycodone (OxyContin)

   b. Meperidine (Demerol)

   c. Ibuprofen (Advil)

   d. Acetaminophen (Tylenol)

33. Why are selective COX-2 inhibitors often prescribed over aspirin?

   a. They are more effective at relieving severe pain.

   b. They are more effective at relieving dull, throbbing pain.

   c. They are less expensive.

   d. They cause fewer side effects.

34. ASA is an abbreviation that refers to which of the following?

   a. Any NSAID

   b. Aspirin

   c. Opioid analgesics

   d. COX-2 inhibitors

35. A healthcare provider sees an order for aspirin 325 mg once daily. The healthcare provider knows this medication is given at this dose level for what reason?

   a. To prolong clotting times

   b. To fight infections

   c. To relieve pain

   d. To decrease inflammation

36. When a healthcare provider is asked to explain why Tylenol is used more often than aspirin, the response is that aspirin can cause which of the following?

   a. Dependence

   b. Increased platelet adhesiveness

   c. GI bleeding

   d. CNS depression

37. A mother asks why aspirin should not be given to children and teens. The appropriate reaction by the healthcare provider is based on the actions of aspirin, which can cause which of the following?

   a. Anticoagulant activity

   b. Reduced incidence of strokes

   c. Reduced risk of colorectal cancer

   d. Increased risk of Reye's syndrome

38. Which of the following drugs is commonly given to heroin addicts during treatment of their drug dependence?

    a. Methadone (Dolophine)

    b. Oxycodone

    c. Morphine

    d. Meperidine (Demerol)

39. Why are opioids often used for pain relief following tooth extractions?

    a. They help the client sleep.

    b. They do not prolong bleeding time.

    c. They can be taken once a day.

    d. They are more efficacious than other analgesics.

40. A healthcare provider knows that therapeutic effects of opiates do not include which of the following?

    a. Treatment of respiratory depression

    b. Treatment of diarrhea

    c. Relief of severe pain

    d. Suppression of cough reflex

41. A client comes to the ER with an overdose of morphine. What would the priority nursing assessment include?

    a. Dilated pupils

    b. Depressed respiration

    c. Hypertension

    d. Diarrhea

42. For an overdose of opiates, what would the healthcare provider need to have on hand to counteract the effects?

    a. Dextroamphetamine (Dexedrine)

    b. Phenytoin (Dilantin)

    c. Naloxone (Narcan)

    d. Tramadol (Ultram)

43. A client comes to the ER with a migraine. The healthcare provider knows that the client may have an aura prior to the onset of the headache. What does the aura indicate about the client?

    a. The client has taken an overdose of aspirin.

    b. The client has taken an overdose of opioids.

    c. The client will soon be experiencing a migraine.

    d. The client has a high fever.

44. What is the mechanism of action of sumatriptan (Imitrex) and other triptans?

    a. Affect mu receptors

    b. Cause vasoconstriction of cranial arteries

c. Block prostaglandin synthesis

d. Block COX-2

MAKING CONNECTIONS

45. Besides an antimigraine agent, what is another use for amitriptyline?

a. Anticonvulsant

b. Sedative hypnotic

c. Antipsychotic

d. Antidepressant

46. Ergotamine is a Category X drug, which means what about the drug?

a. Has a high risk of physical and psychological dependence

b. Should never be taken during pregnancy

c. Has no therapeutic use

d. Is very toxic to the client

47. Phenobarbital (Luminal) is a sedative-hypnotic that is also prescribed for which of the following?

a. Migraines

b. Marijuana addiction

c. Seizures

d. Clinical depression

48. Where would an intrathecal injection of morphine be administered?

a. Spinal subarachnoid space

b. Brain

c. Joint

d. Abdominal cavity

49. What is the first step in pharmacokinetics?

a. Metabolism

b. Absorption

c. Ingestion

d. Excretion

CALCULATIONS

50. The physician orders ibuprofen 400 mg PO tid. The pharmacy sends ibuprofen suspension 100 mg/5 ml. The client should receive _____ml per dose.

51. The physician orders naloxone HCL 0.4 mg IV bolus now. The pharmacy supplies naloxone 0.02 mg/ml. The nurse should administer _____ml IV bolus now.

CASE STUDY APPLICATIONS

52. Mr. T arrives in your office complaining of severe pain in his joints. You are asked to assess this client's complaints and recommend a course of treatment. He is 75 years old and, other than anxiety and insomnia, appears to be in good health. Mr. T is interested in nonpharmacologic control of his pain. He admits to being reluctant to take the oxycodone that the physician ordered, because he does not want to "become a crazy addict." The nurse has chosen knowledge deficit for a nursing diagnosis.

    a. What interventions would be appropriate for this situation?

    b. What outcomes would be evaluated for this patient?

53. Ms. M has been experiencing migraine headaches for 2 years. She is now seeking medical assistance because they have become more frequent and painful. She states that it takes six aspirin to relieve the pain once the migraine has started. She has a history of chronic heart failure and hypertension. She has heard that drugs used for migraines are addictive and is interested in a nonpharmacologic solution. The following medications are being taken:

    Oxycodone terephthalate (Percodan) (as needed)

    Verapamil (Calan)

    Digoxin (Lanoxin)

    a. The nurse chooses "altered comfort: pain" as the diagnosis. What interventions can be used for this nursing diagnosis?

    b. What patient goals would be included in the care for this patient?

CHAPTER 20

DRUGS FOR LOCAL AND GENERAL ANESTHESIA

OBJECTIVES

To view the objectives, please refer to the textbook, student CD-ROM, and the Companion Website at *www.prenhall.com/adams*.

FILL IN THE BLANK

From the textbook, find the correct word(s) to complete the statement(s).

1. Because local anesthesia is not always applied to small areas of the body, some local anesthetic treatments are more accurately called _____ anesthesia.

2. The direct injection of a local anesthetic into tissue immediate to a surgical site is called _____ anesthesia.

3. The goal of general anesthesia is to provide a rapid and complete loss of _____.

4. The two major ways to induce general anesthesia are by using _____ agents and _____ agents.

5. Opioids are sometimes given as preoperative medications to counteract _____ .

6. Local anesthesia is loss of _____ to a small area without loss of _____.

7. In applying local anesthesia, the method employed depends on _____ and _____.

8. In the area where the local anesthetic is applied, _____ and _____ will temporarily diminish.

9. Drug classes used as adjuncts to anesthesia include _____, _____, _____, and _____.

10. The advantage of _____ anesthesia is that the dose of anesthetic can be _____, thus making the procedure safer for the patient.

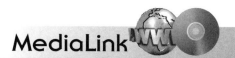

MediaLink

www.prenhall.com/adams

CD-ROM
Animation:
   Mechanism in Action: Lidocaine
   (Xylocaine)
Audio Glossary
NCLEX Review

Companion Website
NCLEX Review
Dosage Calculations
Case Study
Care Plans
Expanded Key Concepts

MATCHING

For questions 11 through 23, match the drug in column I with its classification in column II.

Column I	Column II
11. _____ Droperidol (Inapsine)	a. Ester-type local anesthetic
12. _____ Benzocaine (Anbesol)	b. Amide-type local anesthetic
13. _____ Bupivacaine (Marcaine)	c. Inhaled anesthetic
14. _____ Enflurane (Ethrane)	d. Intravenous anesthetic
15. _____ Diazepam (Valium)	e. Adjunct to anesthesia
16. _____ Lidocaine (Xylocaine)	
17. _____ Prilocaine (Citanest)	
18. _____ Fentanyl (Duragesic, Actiq, others)	
19. _____ Promethazine (Phenergan, others)	
20. _____ Ketamine (Ketalar)	
21. _____ Isoflurane (Forane)	
22. _____ Pentobarbital (Nembutal)	
23. _____ Thiopental (Pentothal)	

For questions 24 through 32, match the characteristics in column I with their drugs or classes in column II.

Column I	Column II
24. _____ Prolongs duration of local anesthetic agents	a. Epinephrine
25. _____ Most commonly used topical anesthetics	b. Epidural
26. _____ May be prescribed for cardiac dysrhythmias	c. Amides
27. _____ Type of anesthesia most commonly used in OB during labor and delivery	d. Benzocaine
28. _____ Most commonly used injectable local anesthetic	e. Lidocaine
29. _____ Most commonly used local anesthetic	f. Isoflurane (Forane)
30. _____ Most abused anesthetic agent	g. Succinylcholine
31. _____ Major depolarizing neuromuscular blocker	h. Nitrous oxide
32. _____ Most widely used inhalation anesthesia	

MULTIPLE CHOICE

33. Epinephrine is often added to a local anesthetic. The nurse must monitor for which factors when caring for the patient who is due to receive epinephrine in his anesthetic?

    a. Side effects of increased heart rate and BP

    b. History of cardiac conditions

    c. Vital signs

    d. All of the above

34. Which of the following is *not* a major route for applying local anesthetics?

    a. Epidural

    b. Spinal

    c. Nerve block

    d. Inhalation

35. In administering general anesthetics using balanced anesthesia, the nurse would expect which medication to be administered first?

    a. IV anesthesia

    b. Inhalation anesthesia

    c. Analgesics

    d. Neuromuscular blocking agents

36. Nitrous oxide can be administered safely in patients with which of the following?

    a. Myasthenia gravis

    b. Increased anxiety related to pain or procedures

    c. Increased intracranial pressure

    d. Cardiac disease

37. An alkaline substance such as sodium hydroxide is sometimes added to a vial of anesthetic solution for what reason?

    a. To provide the environment needed for absorption

    b. To prolong the duration of anesthetic action

    c. To increase the effectiveness of the anesthetic in regions that have extensive local infection or abscesses

    d. To decrease the potential for anaphylaxis

38. Which of the following is a potential early adverse effect from local anesthetics?

    a. Hypertension

    b. Myocardial infarction

    c. Flushing

    d. Restlessness or anxiety

39. Which stage of general anesthesia is called surgical anesthesia because it is the stage in which most surgery occurs?

    a. Stage 1

    b. Stage 2

    c. Stage 3

    d. Stage 4

40. The *primary* reason why nitrous oxide is used in dentistry is it provides which of the following?

    a. Potent analgesia

    b. Sedation/relaxation

    c. Anti-inflammatory properties

    d. Anti-infective properties

41. Inhaled general anesthetics produce their affect by preventing the flow of which of the following into neurons of the CNS.

    a. Carbohydrates

    b. Lipids

    c. Sodium

    d. Calcium

42. Which of the following is a potential early adverse effect from nitrous oxide?

    a. Restlessness or anxiety

    b. Dysrhythmia

    c. Hypertension

    d. Mania

43. What is the major depolarizing neuromuscular blocker used during surgery?

    a. Succinylcholine (Anectine)

    b. Acetylcholine

    c. Promethazine (Phenergan)

    d. Bethanechol (Urecholine)

44. Which of the following is a parasympathomimetic sometimes administered to stimulate the smooth muscle of the bowel and the urinary tract following surgery?

    a. Succinylcholine (Anectine)

    b. Acetylcholine

    c. Promethazine (Phenergan)

    d. Bethanechol (Urecholine)

45. Halothane hepatitis can be prevented by using Halothane?

    a. in those presently not pregnant

    b. at least 21 days apart

    c. with caution in those having diminished hepatic function

    d. with in those having high blood pressure or irregular heart beats

MAKING CONNECTIONS

46. In addition to its use as an injected anesthetic, what is lorazepam (Ativan) also used to treat?

    a. Depression

    b. Anxiety

    c. Loss of appetite

    d. Bipolar disorder

47. Where are sublingual medications administered?

    a. Into a body cavity

    b. Into the subarachnoid spinal space

    c. Into a vein or artery

    d. Under the tongue

48. Which of the following is a hallucinogen?

    a. Psilocybin

    b. Cocaine

    c. Heroin

    d. Marijuana

49. Before administering an opioid, which of the following should be checked?

    a. Blood pressure

    b. Respiration rate

    c. Body temperature

    d. Pulse rate

50. Adrenergic blockers produce a response similar to that of which of the following?

    a. Sympathetic stimulation

    b. Parasympathetic stimulation

    c. Dopaminergic inhibition

    d. Serotonin inhibition

CALCULATIONS

51. Atropine grains 1/6 SC is ordered. Availability is 15 mg/ml. How many milliliters would be given?

52. Trimethobenzamide (Tigan) 100 mg is ordered IM stat.
    Availability is an ampule with 200 mg/2 cc. How many milliliters would be given?

CASE STUDY APPLICATIONS

53. Ms. K is to undergo a procedure that requires general anesthesia. She asks the nurse what to expect from the medications and before and after the procedure.

   a. Identify the nursing diagnosis.

   b. Describe interventions that would be appropriate for this patient.

54. Mrs. B is to have a minor procedure on her foot during which local anesthesia is to be used. She is anxious and asks how this procedure is done. She asks what type of effect the anesthesia will have and how long the anesthesia will last. Mrs. B has rapid speech and talks in a pressured speech pattern. She is tremulous and seems to be restless, scanning the room frequently.

   a. Identify the nursing diagnosis.

   b. What assessment data would cause the nurse to have picked this diagnosis?

   c. Describe interventions that would be appropriate for this patient.

   d. Identify the goal(s) for this patient.

   e. How would each goal be evaluated by the nurse?

CHAPTER 21

DRUGS FOR HYPERTENSION

OBJECTIVES

To view the objectives, please refer to the textbook, student CD-ROM, and the Companion Website at *www.prenhall.com/adams*.

FILL IN THE BLANK

From the textbook, find the correct word(s) to complete the statement(s).

1. The most common type of hypertension, accounting for 90% of all cases, is called _____ hypertension.

2. As cardiac output increases, the blood pressure _____.

3. Angiotensin II raises blood pressure by _____.

4. Calcium channel blockers cause the smooth muscle in arterioles to_____ , thus_____ blood pressure.

5. ACE inhibitors such as captopril (Capoten) reduce blood pressure by lowering levels of _____ and _____.

6. _____ is a condition that occurs when the heart rate increases due to the rapid fall in blood pressure created by a drug.

7. The side effects of adrenergic blockers are generally quite predictable, since they are usually extensions of the _____ response.

8. _____ are found in the aorta and internal carotid. They act as sensors for the vascular system.

9. When the heart is not ejecting blood, the pressure in the arteries is called _____ blood pressure.

10. _____ are often the first-line medications for the treatment of hypertension.

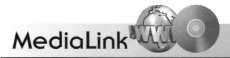

MediaLink

www.prenhall.com/adams

CD-ROM
Animations:
    Mechanism in Action: Nifedipine (Procordia)
    Mechanism in Action: Doxazosin (Cardura)
Audio Glossary
NCLEX Review
Companion Website
NCLEX Review
Dosage Calculations
Case Study
Care Plans
Expanded Key Concepts

MATCHING

For questions 11 through 20, match the drug in column I with its pharmacologic classification in column II.

Column I		Column II
11. _____ Clonidine (Catapres)		a. Diuretic
12. _____ Captopril (Capoten)		b. Calcium channel blocker
13. _____ Spironolactone (Aldactone)		c. ACE inhibitor or angiotensin receptor blocker
14. _____ Diltiazem (Cardizem)		d. Beta$_1$-blocker
15. _____ Losartan (Cozaar)		e. Alpha$_1$-blocker
16. _____ Verapamil (Calan)		f. Centrally acting alpha$_2$ agonist
17. _____ Lisinopril (Prinivil)		g. Direct vasodilator
18. _____ Hydralazine (Apresoline)		
19. _____ Metoprolol (Toprol)		
20. _____ Hydrochlorothiazide (HydroDIURIL)		

MULTIPLE CHOICE

21. Which of the following lowers blood pressure primarily by increasing the renal excretion of sodium and water?

    a. Doxazosin (Cardura)

    b. Furosemide (Lasix)

    c. Verapamil (Calan)

    d. Quinapril (Accupril)

22. Which of the following is a cardioselective beta$_1$-blocker?

    a. Propranolol (Inderal)

    b. Doxazosin (Cardura)

    c. Ipratropium (Atrovent)

    d. Atenolol (Tenormin)

23. The nurse takes a patient's blood pressure at 157/83 mm Hg. In a patient over age 80, what is this considered?

    a. Reason to begin diuretic therapy

    b. Reason to begin aggressive therapy with furosemide (Lasix)

    c. Normal

    d. Reason to begin therapy with sympatholytics

24. Which of the following is *not* a primary factor responsible for blood pressure?

    a. Venous pressure

    b. Cardiac output

    c. Resistance of the small arteries

    d. Blood volume

25. As it relates to antihypertensive therapy, what is stepped care?

    a. Two or more drugs from the same class

    b. Two or more drugs from different classes

    c. One drug during weeks 1 to 3, then a new drug starting in week 4

    d. One week of drug therapy alternating with 1 week of no drug administration

26. Which drug class is *not* commonly used to treat hypertension?

    a. Calcium channel blockers

    b. Angiotensin-converting enzyme inhibitors

    c. Direct-acting vasodilators

    d. Sodium channel blockers

27. Which drugs are first-line drugs for treating mild to moderate hypertension because they act on the kidney tubule to block reabsorption of sodium?

    a. Diuretics

    b. Calcium channel blockers

    c. Direct vasodilators

    d. Alpha-blockers

28. The nurse should carefully monitor for hyperkalemia when patients are taking which drug?

    a. Diuretics

    b. Calcium channel blockers

    c. Direct vasodilators

    d. Alpha-blockers

29. Calcium channel blockers used for hypertension act by blocking calcium ion channels in which of the following?

    a. Skeletal muscle

    b. Vascular smooth muscle

    c. Central nervous system

    d. Kidney

30. Which drug class will stimulate the secretion of aldosterone?

    a. Diuretics

    b. Calcium channel blockers

    c. ACE inhibitors

    d. Alpha-blockers

31. Which of the following types of drugs are used to treat hypertension?

    a. Sympathomimetics

    b. Selective beta$_1$-blockers

    c. Selective beta$_2$-blockers

    d. Parasympathomimetics

32. The nurse should carefully monitor for bradycardia in patients taking which of the following?

    a. Selective beta1-blockers

    b. Calcium channel blockers

    c. ACE inhibitors

    d. Alpha-blockers

33. Which of the following would be used to lower extremely high blood pressure within minutes?

    a. Hydralazine (Apresoline)

    b. Nitroprusside (Nitropress)

    c. Doxazosin (Cardura)

    d. Prazosin (Minipress)

34. In response to falling blood pressure, what does the kidney release?

    a. Renin

    b. Aldosterone

    c. Angiotensin

    d. Potassium

35. In asthmatic patients, the nurse should monitor carefully for signs and symptoms of bronchoconstriction when using which class of antihypertensives?

    a. Alpha-blockers

    b. Calcium channel blockers

    c. ACE inhibitors

    d. Beta-blockers

MAKING CONNECTIONS

36. Which drug or drug class is *not* given to prevent thrombi formation?

    a. Thrombolytics

    b. Aspirin

    c. Heparin

    d. Warfarin

37. Which of the following routes for hydromorphone should be used to achieve the most rapid onset of action?

    a. PO 8.0 mg

    b. SC 1.5 mg

    c. IV 0.80 mg

    d. Rectal 3.0 mg

38. For hypertension, the nurse administers an average daily dose of 5.0 mg for enalapril and 10.0 mg for fosinopril. From this information, what may the nurse correctly conclude?

    a. Enalapril is twice as efficacious as fosinopril.

b. Enalapril will likely produce fewer side effects than fosinopril.

c. Enalapril is more potent than fosinopril.

d. The onset of action for fosinopril will take longer than that of enalapril.

39. Atropine is a prototype for which drug class?

a. Sympathomimetics

b. Beta-adrenergic blockers

c. Parasympathomimetics

d. Cholinergic blockers

40. Which of the following drugs is often combined in cartridges with local anesthetics?

a. Epinephrine

b. Atropine

c. Heparin

d. Acetaminophen

CALCULATIONS

41. Furosemide 15 mg is ordered. The bottle reads: 20 mg/2 ml. How much furosemide will the nurse draw up in the syringe?

42. Your cardiac patient has Cardizem 60 mg qid ordered. How many tablets will the nurse administer if the bottle reads diltiazem HCl (Cardizem) 120 mg/tablet?

CASE STUDY APPLICATIONS

43. Mr. H, age 50, has presented a blood pressure of 170/100 mm Hg the last two visits to his doctor. Hydrochlorothiazide (HydroDIURIL) was prescribed for him about 1 year ago. Other than some anxiety, he offers no complaints and other vital signs are normal. His blood lipids are elevated, he is 20 pounds overweight, and he smokes a pack of cigarettes a day; otherwise he appears healthy.

a. What assessment data help you understand the contributing factors for Mr. H's hypertension?

b. You suspect that Mr. H has not been taking his medication. What nursing diagnoses would you identify? What outcomes would you select for the diagnoses?

c. Assuming Mr. H has been taking his HydroDIURIL, what is the next logical pharmacologic option for him?

44. Ms. F is a 75-year-old patient who has been taking enalapril (Vasotec) and chlorothiazide for hypertension for the past 2 years. She is very compliant, taking walks daily, watching her salt intake, and eating plenty of potassium-rich foods such as bananas. Two weeks ago, her physician increased her dose of enalapril and switched her to spironolactone instead of chlorothiazide. She is now in the office complaining that she gets dizzy and falls over every morning when she gets out of bed, and that she feels like her heart is racing when she walks. Although her blood pressure is normal, she wants to be switched back to her previous medications.

a. What assessment data lead you to understand the potential cause of her dizziness? What teaching might be done to help solve this problem?

b. An ECG on Ms. F is normal. Can you recognize anything in her history that might be responsible for her heart complaints? What assessment information would help you define her problem?

c. Is it necessary to change Ms. F's medication or is it possible that her complaints could be resolved through patient teaching?

CHAPTER 22

DRUGS FOR HEART FAILURE

OBJECTIVES

To view the objectives, please refer to the textbook, student CD-ROM, and the Companion Website at *www.prenhall.com/adams*.

FILL IN THE BLANK

From the textbook, find the correct word(s) to complete the statement(s).

1. The resting phase of the cardiac cycle between beats is known as the _____.

2. As more stretch is applied to myocardial fibers, they will contract with greater force. This is known as the _____ law.

3. As a general rule, if the heart rate is less than _____ beats per minute, digoxin (Lanoxin) should not be taken.

4. Heart failure is an inability of the ventricles to _____ blood.

5. The two most important variables that affect cardiac output are _____ and _____.

6. Engorgement of the liver and peripheral edema is most likely to occur in _____ heart failure.

7. When a medication has a positive inotropic effect, it has the ability to _____ the _____ of the myocardial contraction.

8. Cardiac glycosides cause the heart to beat more _____ and more _____.

9. If a patient has taken an overdose of digoxin, the nurse will prepare to give _____ to treat this life-threatening problem.

10. Blocking phosphodiesterase has the effect of _____ the amount of calcium available for myocardial contraction.

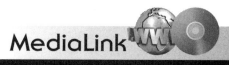

MediaLink

www.prenhall.com/adams

CD-ROM
Animations:
  Mechanism in Action: Digoxin (Lanaxin)
  Mechanism in Action: Lisinopril (Prinuil)
  Mechanism in Action: Furosemide (Lasix)
Audio Glossary
NCLEX Review
Companion Website
NCLEX Review
Dosage Calculations
Case Study
Care Plans
Expanded Key Concepts

MATCHING

For questions 11 through 21, match the drug in column I with its classification in column II.

<table>
<tr><td colspan="2">Column I</td><td>Column II</td></tr>
<tr><td>11. _____</td><td>Lisinopril (Prinivil)</td><td>a. Diuretic</td></tr>
<tr><td>12. _____</td><td>Hydralazine (Apresoline)</td><td>b. Cardiac glycoside</td></tr>
<tr><td>13. _____</td><td>Carvedilol (Coreg)</td><td>c. ACE inhibitor</td></tr>
<tr><td>14. _____</td><td>Hydrochlorothiazide (HydroDIURIL)</td><td>d. Beta-blocker</td></tr>
<tr><td>15. _____</td><td>Milrinone (Primacor)</td><td>e. Direct vasodilator</td></tr>
<tr><td>16. _____</td><td>Amrinone (Inocor)</td><td>f. Phosphodiesterase inhibitor</td></tr>
<tr><td>17. _____</td><td>Quinapril (Accupril)</td><td></td></tr>
<tr><td>18. _____</td><td>Triamterene (Dyrenium)</td><td></td></tr>
<tr><td>19. _____</td><td>Enalapril (Vasotec)</td><td></td></tr>
<tr><td>20. _____</td><td>Isosorbide dinitrate (Isordil)</td><td></td></tr>
<tr><td>21. _____</td><td>Digoxin (Lanoxin)</td><td></td></tr>
</table>

MULTIPLE CHOICE

22. The primary action of digoxin (Lanoxin) that makes it very effective at treating heart failure is its ability to do which of the following?

    a. Dilate the coronary arteries

    b. Increase impulse conduction across the myocardium

    c. Decrease blood pressure

    d. Increase cardiac contractility/output

23. Blood electrolyte levels are critical to safe digoxin therapy. The nurse must carefully monitor for which of the following, which significantly reduces the effectiveness of digoxin?

    a. Hypokalemia

    b. Hyperkalemia

    c. Hypocalcemia

    d. Hypercalcemia

24. What is the best definition of heart failure?

    a. Enlargement of the heart

    b. Inability of the heart to beat in a coordinated manner

    c. Inability of the ventricles to pump sufficient blood

    d. Congestion in the lungs caused by damage to the myocardium

25. What is the amount of blood pumped by each ventricle per minute called?

    a. Preload

    b. Afterload

    c. Stroke volume

    d. Cardiac output

26. What is the correct definition of preload?

    a. Amount of blood pumped by each ventricle per minute

    b. Degree to which the heart fibers are stretched just prior to contraction

    c. Pressure in the aorta that must be overcome for blood to be ejected from the heart

    d. Ability to increase the strength of contraction

27. Which of the following drug classes was first derived from the common plant known as the purple foxglove?

    a. Cardiac glycosides

    b. ACE inhibitors

    c. Phosphodiesterase inhibitors

    d. Beta-adrenergic blockers

28. When monitoring patients on cardiac glycosides, the nurse knows that these drugs help the heart to beat more forcefully and which of the following?

    a. With a faster heart rate

    b. With a slower heart rate

    c. Do not affect cardiac output

    d. With a diminished cardiac output

29. Digoxin (Lanoxin) acts by which of the following?

    a. Blocking beta-adrenergic receptors in the heart

    b. Stimulating beta-adrenergic receptors in the heart

    c. Inhibiting Na^+-K^+ ATPase

    d. Stimulating Na^+-K^+ ATPase

30. The nurse should monitor for which of the following adverse effects in a patient taking digoxin for HF?

    a. Increased heart rate

    b. Increased cardiac output

    c. Increased urine production

    d. Decreased peripheral edema

31. What is potentially the most serious adverse effect of pharmacotherapy with digoxin?

    a. Permanent visual disturbances

    b. Hyperkalemia

    c. Hypotension

    d. Dysrhythmias

32. Which drug class has largely replaced the cardiac glycosides as first-line drugs in the therapy of heart failure?

    a. Direct vasodilators

    b. ACE inhibitors

    c. Phosphodiesterase inhibitors

    d. Beta-adrenergic blockers

33. The primary action of the ACE inhibitors that benefits a patient with HF is a decrease in which of the following?

    a. Peripheral resistance/blood pressure

    b. Cardiac output

    c. Heart rate

    d. Urine output

34. By what mechanism does isosorbide dinitrate (Isordil) benefit patients with HF?

    a. Lowering arterial blood pressure

    b. Increasing urine output

    c. Reducing venous return, causing a decrease in cardiac workload

    d. Slowing the heart rate, causing a reduction in cardiac workload

35. In addition to heart failure, what is hydralazine (Apresoline) also prescribed for?

    a. Coagulation disorders

    b. Hypertension

    c. Stroke

    d. Glaucoma

36. In addition to heart failure, what are diuretics also commonly prescribed for?

    a. Minor depression

    b. Coagulation disorders

    c. Hypertension

    d. Dysrhythmias

37. By what mechanism do diuretics such as furosemide (Lasix) improve the symptoms of heart failure?

    a. Blockading beta-adrenergic receptors

    b. Causing the heart to beat with more strength

    c. Reducing fluid/plasma volume

    d. Slowing heart rate, thus reducing cardiac workload

38. The nurse must carefully monitor for which of the following serious side effects of furosemide therapy?

    a. Electrolyte imbalances

    b. Dysrhythmias

    c. Reflex tachycardia

    d. Hypertension

39. What is the primary use of the phosphodiesterase inhibitors in HF patients?

    a. Cause a rapid reduction in fluid/plasma volume

    b. Cause the heart to beat faster

    c. Rapidly lower blood pressure

    d. Increase the force of contraction and increase cardiac output

40. How may beta-adrenergic blockers such as carvedilol (Coreg) improve HF?

    a. Increase heart rate

    b. Decrease heart rate

    c. Cause the heart to contract with more force

    d. Lower blood pressure and reduce cardiac workload

MAKING CONNECTIONS

41. Which of the following classes of drugs is *not* used for hypertension?

    a. Sodium channel blockers

    b. ACE inhibitors

    c. Adrenergic blockers

    d. Diuretics

42. The nurse should teach patients to eat plenty of bananas during pharmacotherapy with thiazide diuretics, to get a sufficient supply of which of the following?

    a. Selenium

    b. Calcium

    c. Potassium

    d. Chloride

43. The nurse is asked to administer carvedilol 6.25 mg bid. What does the term *bid* mean?

    a. Twice a week

    b. Twice a day

    c. Before bedtime

    d. Before breakfast

44. Which of the following is *not* a drug class that has significant potential for abuse by patients?

    a. Barbiturates

    b. Benzodiazepines

c. Opioids

d. Anticholinergic

45. Which drug class is used to dry secretions, treat asthma, and prevent motion sickness?

   a. Anticholinergics

   b. Cholinergics

   c. Parasympathomimetics

   d. Alpha-blockers

CALCULATIONS

46. A solution of amrinone lactate 100 mg in 40 ml NS is ordered to infuse at 5 mcg/kg/min for a patient weighing 75 kg. What is the ml/hr flow rate?

47. A doctor orders furosemide 40 mg IV push. The bottle label reads: Furosimide 20 mg/2 ml. How many milliliters will the nurse give?

CASE STUDY APPLICATIONS

48. Drugs can affect the heart in a number of ways. It is essential that the nurse understand the underlying cardiac pathophysiology in order to understand drug action.

   a. Explain the difference between an inotropic effect and a chronotropic effect.

   b. Give examples of pharmacologic classes of drugs that affect each.

   c. In general, is it more desirable to give a drug with a positive inotropic effect or a positive chronotropic effect when treating chronic heart failure? Explain your answer.

49. Mr. L has just been diagnosed with early heart failure and his physician has prescribed hydrochlorothiazide (HydroDIURIL), atorvastatin (Lipitor), and lisinopril (Prinivil). His blood pressure is slightly elevated, his blood cholesterol is marginally high, and he has stenosis of the mitral valve that seems to be worsening. Although he is not an athletic person, Mr. L likes to take long walks after dinner. He confides that at his age of 60 he has no intention of taking any of the medications, but intends to try Chinese herbal therapy.

   a. You are developing a teaching plan for Mr. L. You want to explain the rationale for each of his medications. What information will you include in the teaching plan?

   b. How do you assess Mr. L's need for alternative therapy, and what is your best response to his concern about prescription drugs?

   c. Knowing that health promotion is an essential nursing action, what lifestyle changes would you suggest to Mr. L to improve his cardiac health?

50. Mrs. C, an elderly patient, is transferred from a rehabilitation center to an acute care setting with a diagnosis of heart failure and the following vital signs: BP 120/90, pulse 108/min, and labored respiration 32/min. Assessment of breath sounds reveals coarse rhonchi and wheezing on inspiration and expiration. A 10-pound weight gain has been observed over a 3-day period. The care plan includes digoxin 0.5 mg IV STAT to be repeated in 4 hours and then an oral dose of 0.25 mg/day.

   a. What assessment data support the diagnosis of heart failure?

   b. Why would the care plan include a STAT dose of digoxin with a dose repeating in 4 hours and then a lower daily dose?

   c. What other bodily system must the nurse pay close attention to in the assessment of this patient with heart failure?

CHAPTER 23

DRUGS FOR DYSRHYTHMIAS

OBJECTIVES

To view the objectives, please refer to the textbook, student CD-ROM, and the Companion Website at *www.prenhall.com/adams*.

FILL IN THE BLANK

From the textbook, find the correct word(s) to complete the statement(s).

1. After the action potential has passed and the myocardial cell is in a depolarized state, repolarization depends on removal of

   _____ from the cell.

2. Calcium channel blockers are only effective against

   _____ dysrhythmias.

3. Severe dysrhythmias may result in _____.

4. Dysrhythmias that originate in the atria are sometimes referred to as _____.

5. The most common type of dysrhythmia is _____.

6. The SA node is also called the _____ of the heart.

7. Electrical shock of the heart to treat a dysrhythmia is called _____.

8. The adverse vascular effect related to the use of quinidine is _____.

9. Beta-blockers are contraindicated for patients with three types of heart abnormalities:_____ ,

   _____, and _____.

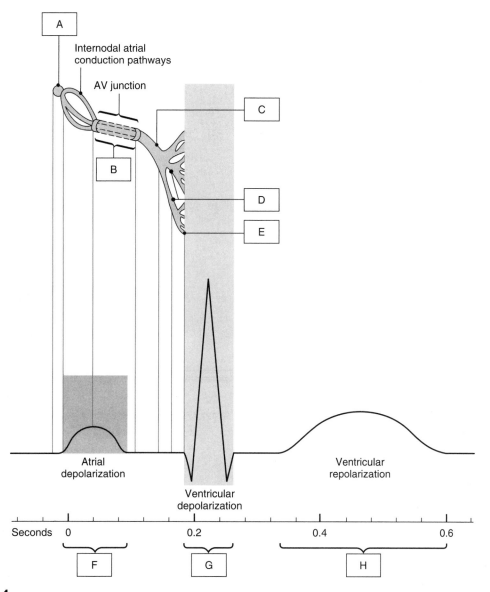

Figure 23–1

SOURCE: Core Concepts in Pharmacology, Workbook by Holland/Adams © 2003. Reprinted by permission of Pearson Education, Inc., Upper Saddle River, NJ.

10. Label the parts of the conduction pathway and the events of the ECG in Figure 23–1.

   a. _____

   b. _____

   c. _____

   d. _____

   e. _____

   f. _____

   g. _____

   h. _____

MATCHING

For questions 11 through 21, match the drug in column I with its classification in column II.

Column I	**Column II**
11. _____ Quinidine gluconate (Duraquin)	a. Sodium channel blocker
12. _____ Esmolol (Brevibloc)	b. Potassium channel blocker
13. _____ Amiodarone (Cordarone)	c. Beta-adrenergic blocker
14. _____ Diltiazem (Cardizem)	d. Calcium channel blocker
15. _____ Verapamil (Calan)	e. Miscellaneous (none of the above)
16. _____ Phenytoin (Dilantin)	
17. _____ Propranolol (Inderal)	
18. _____ Lidocaine (Xylocaine)	
19. _____ Procainamide (Pronestyl)	
20. _____ Adenosine (Adenocard)	
21. _____ Disopyramide (Norpace)	

MULTIPLE CHOICE

22. Which of the following best describes dysrhythmias?

    a. Abnormalities of electrical conduction in the heart

    b. Diminished cardiac output

    c. Narrowing of the coronary arteries

    d. High blood pressure

23. Which of the following is *not* a type of dysrhythmia?

    a. Atrial tachycardia

    b. Ventricular flutter

    c. Sinus bradycardia

    d. Premature subventricular contractions

24. Where do electrical impulses in the heart generally begin?

    a. Atrioventricular bundle

    b. Atrioventricular (AV) node

    c. Sinoatrial (SA) node

    d. Purkinje fibers

25. Under resting conditions, a new action potential crosses the myocardium approximately how many times every minute?

    a. 60

    b. 75

c. 85

d. 110

26. In most myocardial cells and in neurons, an action potential begins when channels located in the plasma membrane open and _____ rushes into the cell, producing a rapid depolarization.

    a. Calcium

    b. Phosphate

    c. Potassium

    d. Sodium

27. Which of the following is *not* a class of antidysrhythmic drugs?

    a. Sodium channel blockers

    b. Alpha-adrenergic blockers

    c. Potassium channel blockers

    d. Calcium channel blockers

28. Which of the following is the basic pharmacologic mechanism by which nearly all antidysrhythmic drugs terminate or prevent abnormal rhythms?

    a. Increase heart rate until rhythm returns to normal

    b. Dilate coronary arteries so that more blood gets to the myocardium

    c. Slow the impulse conduction velocity until rhythm returns to normal

    d. Lower the blood pressure so the heart has less workload

29. A blockade of sodium channels in myocardial cells will do which of the following?

    a. Slow the spread of impulse conduction

    b. Speed the spread of impulse conduction

    c. Stop the spread of impulse conduction

    d. Worsen a dysrhythmia

30. Lidocaine is given _____ to terminate _____ dysrhythmias.

    a. PO, ventricular

    b. PO, atria

    c. IV, atrial

    d. IV, ventricular

31. Which antidysrhythmic drug acts by blocking beta-adrenergic receptors in the heart?

    a. Verapamil (Calan)

    b. Digoxin (Lanoxin)

    c. Amiodarone (Cordarone)

    d. Propranolol (Inderal)

32. Which of the following is a sodium channel blocker that is the oldest antidysrhythmic drug?

    a. Propranolol (Inderal)

    b. Amiodarone (Cordarone)

    c. Quinidine sulfate (Quinidex)

    d. Verapamil (Calan)

33. The most common side effects of quinidine are related to which body system?

    a. CNS

    b. Gastrointestinal

    c. Cardiovascular

    d. Pulmonary

34. Beta-adrenergic blockers are used to treat a large number of cardiovascular diseases. Which of the following is *not* one of the uses of beta-blockers?

    a. Anticoagulant

    b. Hypertension

    c. Heart failure

    d. Dysrhythmias

35. How do beta-adrenergic blockers prevent dysrhythmias?

    a. Speed impulse conduction across the myocardium

    b. Slow impulse conduction across the myocardium

    c. Blockade calcium channels

    d. Blockade sodium channels

36. Propranolol (Inderal) is classified as which of the following?

    a. Nonselective alpha-and beta-blocker

    b. Nonselective beta-blocker

    c. Selective beta$_1$-blocker

    d. Selective beta$_2$-blocker

37. Which of the following is *not* an expected adverse effect in a patient taking propranolol (Inderal)?

    a. Diminished sex drive

    b. Hypotension

    c. Bradycardia

    d. Tachycardia

38. How do potassium channel blockers prevent dysrhythmias?

    a. Block beta-adrenergic receptors in the myocardium

    b. Reduce blood pressure

    c. Interfere with calcium ion channels

    d. Prolong the refractory period of the heart

39. Which potassium channel blocker has become a drug of choice for the treatment of atrial dysrhythmias in patients with heart failure?

    a. Bretylium (Bretylol)

    b. Dofetilide (Tikosyn)

    c. Amiodarone (Cordarone)

    d. Sotalol (Betapace)

40. The most serious adverse effects from amiodarone (Cordarone) are related to which body system?

    a. CNS

    b. Pulmonary

    c. Cardiovascular

    d. Gastrointestinal

41. Blocking calcium ion channels has a number of effects on the heart and vascular system. These effects are most similar to which of the following?

    a. Sodium channel blockers

    b. Potassium channel blockers

    c. Beta-adrenergic blockers

    d. Cardiac glycosides

42. Which of the following antidysrhythmics is used IV to rapidly terminate serious atrial dysrhythmias?

    a. Adenosine (Adenocard)

    b. Amiodarone (Cordarone)

    c. Propranolol (Inderal)

    d. Verapamil (Calan)

MAKING CONNECTIONS

43. The main benefit of phosphodiesterase inhibitors is in the treatment of which of the following?

    a. Hypertension

    b. Coagulation disorders

    c. Heart failure

    d. Shock

44. Which of the following is the most widely used class of agents for the treatment of clinical depression?

    a. Barbiturates

    b. Na^+-K^+ ATPase inhibitors

    c. Benzodiazepines

    d. Selective serotonin reuptake inhibitors

45. A patient taking sumatriptan (Imitrex) likely suffers from which of the following?

    a. Sleep disorders

    b. Seizures

    c. Migraines

    d. Schizophrenia

46. What is GABA?

    a. Surgical procedure used to help patients who are psychotic

    b. Neurotransmitter

    c. Drug used to treat bipolar disorder

    d. Widely abused hallucinogen

CALCULATIONS

47. A solution of Cardizem 125 mg/100 ml D5W is to infuse at a rate of 20 mg/hr. Calculate the ml/hr flow rate.

48. A patient with atrial fibrillation has amiodarone ordered at 0.5 mg/min. The concentration is amiodarone 900 mg in 250 ml D5W. How many ml/hr should the IV pump be programmed to deliver?

CASE STUDY APPLICATIONS

49. Ms. D, age 67, is brought to the hospital by paramedics after collapsing on the street. She has a history of heart failure and has been taking digoxin and furosemide. The ER physician determines that she is experiencing a myocardial infarction accompanied by severe tachycardia.

    a. The ER nurse should collect what assessment data before propranolol is started?

    b. The patient is also given quinidine. Why would this drug be used? What position should Ms. D be in during this IV administration and why?

    c. The nurse should anticipate what adverse effects from the use of quinidine and propranolol?

50. You are working on a progressive care unit (PCU). The monitor technician tells you that a patient, admitted for chest pain, is demonstrating paroxysmal supraventricular tachycardia. You know the patient has a PRN order for verapamil (Calan) if supraventricular tachycardia occurs.

    a. What nursing assessment must you make before administering Calan?

    b. If the patient will remain on Calan, what patient teaching must be done?

    c. What nursing diagnoses may be identified for this patient?

CHAPTER 24

DRUGS FOR COAGULATION DISORDERS

OBJECTIVES

To view the objectives, please refer to the textbook, student CD-ROM, and the Companion Website at *www.prenhall.com/adams*.

FILL IN THE BLANK

From the textbook, find the correct word(s) to complete the statement(s).

1. Identify steps in the coagulation cascade shown in Figure 24–1.

   a. _____

   b. _____

   c. _____

2. Identify steps in fibrinolysis shown in Figure 24–2.

   a. _____

   b. _____

3. A traveling clot is called an _____.

4. The most commonly prescribed coagulation modifers are the _____.

5. The _____ are a class of drugs that dissolve life-threatening clots.

6. _____ are drugs that inhibit the normal removal of fibrin.

7. Two laboratory tests used to determine the anticoagulation effects of Coumadin are _____ and _____.

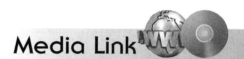

Media Link

www.prenhall.com/adams

CD-ROM
Animation:
   Mechanism in Action: Warfarin (Coumadin)
Audio Glossary
NCLEX Review

Companion Website
NCLEX Review
Dosage Calculations
Case Study
Care Plans
Expanded Key Concepts

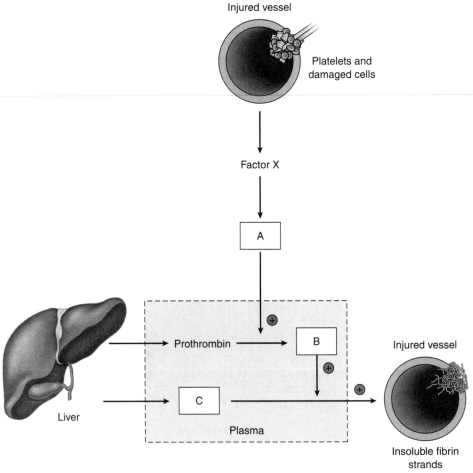

Figure 24–1

SOURCE: Core Concepts in Pharmacology, Workbook by Holland/Adams, © 2003. Reprinted by permission of Pearson Education, Inc., Upper Saddle River, NJ.

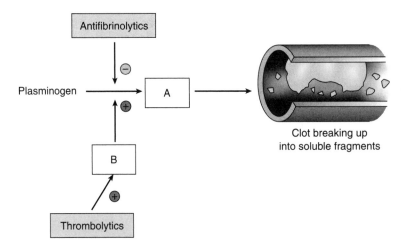

Figure 24–2

SOURCE: Core Concepts in Pharmacology, Workbook by Holland/Adams, © 2003. Reprinted by permission of Pearson Education, Inc., Upper Saddle River, NJ.

MATCHING

For questions 8 through 18, match the drug in column I with its classification in column II.

Column I	Column II
8. _____ Warfarin (Coumadin)	a. Anticoagulant: general type
9. _____ Abciximab (ReoPro)	b. Anticoagulant: antiplatelet type
10. _____ Danaparoid (Orgaran)	c. Anticoagulant: LMWH type
11. _____ Aspirin (ASA)	d. ADP receptor blocker
12. _____ Desmopressin (DDAVP)	e. Glycoprotein IIb/IIIa blocker
13. _____ Enoxaparin (Lovenox)	f. Thrombolytic
14. _____ Alteplase (Activase, t-PA)	g. Antifibrinolytic
15. _____ Reteplase (Retavase)	
16. _____ Tirofiban (Aggrastat)	
17. _____ Aminocaproic acid (Amicar)	
18. _____ Ticlopidine (Ticlid)	

MULTIPLE CHOICE

19. Which of the following clump and adhere to the wall of an injured blood vessel to begin the process of hemostasis?

   a. Platelets

   b. Red blood cells

   c. White blood cells

   d. Antibodies

20. What is the solid, insoluble part of a blood clot called?

   a. Fibrin

   b. Thrombin

   c. Prothrombin

   d. Plasmin

21. Normal blood clotting occurs in about how many minutes?

   a. 2

   b. 3

   c. 6

   d. 10

22. Which organ is responsible for making many of the factors necessary for blood clotting?

   a. Kidney

   b. Liver

   c. Brain

   d. Skin

23. What is the process of clot removal called?

    a. Embolysis

    b. Thrombolysis

    c. Plasminolysis

    d. Fibrinolysis

24. What is the specific class of drugs that promotes the formation of clots called?

    a. Antifibrinolytics

    b. Thrombolytics

    c. Fibrinolytics

    d. Plasminogen activators

25. Which lab test is most commonly used to monitor pharmacotherapy with heparin?

    a. Bleeding time

    b. PT

    c. INR

    d. APTT

26. Anticoagulants are drugs that do which of the following?

    a. Dissolve thrombi that have been recently formed

    b. Shorten PT time

    c. Prevent thrombi from forming or growing larger

    d. Cause platelets to become less sticky

27. What is the primary advantage of using low molecular weight heparins (LMWHs) over heparin?

    a. LMWHs possess greater anticoagulant activity.

    b. LMWHs may be given by the oral route.

    c. LMWHs produce a more stable effect on coagulation, thus fewer lab tests are needed.

    d. LMWHs have a prolonged duration of action.

28. The nurse must monitor for the most serious adverse effect of anticoagulant therapy. Which of the following is the most serious?

    a. Hemorrhage

    b. Severe headaches

    c. Electrolyte depletion

    d. Cardiac arrhythmias

29. The nurse must administer which of the following antagonists, if serious hemorrhage occurs during heparin therapy?

    a. Protamine sulfate

    b. Vitamin K

    c. Adenosine diphosphate (ADP)

    d. Desmopressin (DDAVP)

30. Unlike heparin, the anticoagulant activity of warfarin can take how long to reach its maximum effect?

    a. Several minutes

    b. Several hours

    c. Several days

    d. Several weeks

31. The nurse must ensure that vitamin K is available as an antidote to treat an overdose with which of the following?

    a. Aspirin

    b. Heparin and LMWH

    c. Aminocaproic acid (Amicar)

    d. Warfarin (Coumadin)

32. Upon discontinuation of therapy, how long will the pharmacologic activity of warfarin take to diminish?

    a. 10 minutes

    b. 10 hours

    c. 24 hours

    d. 3 days

33. Aspirin causes its anticoagulant effect by inhibiting which of the following?

    a. Plasminogen

    b. Prothrombin

    c. Thromboxane$_2$

    d. Glycoprotein IIb/IIIa

34. Glycoprotein IIb/IIIa inhibitors act by blocking the final step in which of the following?

    a. Hemostasis

    b. Platelet aggregation

    c. Activation of plasminogen

    d. Formation of vitamin K

35. The primary action of streptokinase is to convert plasminogen to which of the following?

    a. Plasminogen activator

    b. Plasmin

    c. Fibrin

    d. Fibrinogen

36. The nurse understands that the primary action of antifibrinolytics is to do which of the following?

    a. Dissolve thrombi

    b. Prevent thrombi

    c. Reverse the effects of anticoagulants

    d. Prevent excessive bleeding following surgery

37. Which of the following is an antifibrinolytic that is also used to control excessive or nocturnal urination?

    a. Desmopressin (DDAVP)

    b. Abciximab (ReoPro)

    c. Aminocaproic acid (Amicar)

    d. Tranexamic acid (Cyklokapron)

38. Which of the following is *not* an indication for thrombolytic therapy?

    a. Acute myocardial infarction (MI)

    b. Postoperative bleeding

    c. Pulmonary embolism

    d. Deep vein thrombosis (DVT)

MAKING CONNECTIONS

39. A patient is receiving warfarin, which is 98% bound to plasma proteins. The antidepressant paroxetine (Paxil), which is 95% bound, is added to the patient's daily medications. If the paroxetine displaces warfarin from its binding sites, which of the following will most likely occur?

    a. Toxicity to warfarin

    b. Toxicity to paroxetine

    c. Diminished effect from warfarin

    d. Diminished effect from paroxetine

40. The antidepressant imipramine (Tofranil) is metabolized to its active form, desipramine, in the liver. The nurse knows that the dose of imipramine for patients with liver cirrhosis should be which of the following?

    a. Increased above average

    b. Decreased below average

    c. An average dose

    d. This patient should not receive imipramine

41. Which of the following is a widely used class of antipsychotic medications?

    a. Phenothiazines

    b. Benzodiazepines

    c. MAO inhibitors

    d. Anticholinergics

42. What is the primary goal of the nurse for patients experiencing PRN pain medications?

    a. Administer the least amount of pain medication possible

    b. Administer analgesics only when pain becomes intolerable

    c. Ensure that dependence does not develop

    d. Alleviate the pain

43. Of the following four drugs, which is *not* related to the other three?

    a. Phenytoin (Dilantin)

    b. Phenobarbital (Luminal)

    c. Sumatriptan (Imitrex)

    d. Ethosuximide (Zarontin)

CALCULATIONS

44. A patient with deep vein thrombosis has orders for heparin 2500 U per hour. The solution strength is 50,000 U in 1000 ml D5W. Calculate the ml/hr flow rate.

45. A patient is receiving 20,000 U heparin in 500 ml D5W. The rate is set at 30 ml/hr. How many units is the patient receiving per hour? How many units will the patient receive in a day?

CASE STUDY APPLICATIONS

46. Ms. S is being discharged from the hospital following surgery for replacement of a heart valve. She will be placed on long-term warfarin (Coumadin) therapy. You are developing this patient's discharge teaching plan.

    a. List the activities that you will teach Ms. S to avoid.

    b. Describe the signs and symptoms that would alert Ms. S to adverse effects of warfarin therapy.

    c. What medications and what herbal supplements should be avoided while Ms. S is being treated with warfarin?

47. Mr. P, age 50, is being admitted to the hospital for the third time this year. He has a history of alcohol abuse, diabetes, and heart failure. He was brought to the hospital with a complaint of abdominal pain and vomiting of bright red blood. His diagnosis is perforated ulcer. The patient states that he has been taking warfarin for an irregular heartbeat and Glucophage for diabetes.

    a. With this limited admission history, what factors might have contributed to Mr. P's acute bleeding episode?

    b. What nursing diagnoses and patient outcomes would be essential in this situation?

    c. What medications might be ordered for Mr. P?

CHAPTER 25

DRUGS FOR ANGINA PECTORIS, MYOCARDIAL INFARCTION, AND CEREBROVASCULAR ACCIDENT

OBJECTIVES

To view the objectives, please refer to the textbook, student CD-ROM, and the Companion Website at *www.prenhall.com/adams*.

FILL IN THE BLANK

From the textbook, find the correct word(s) to complete the statement(s).

1. Acute chest pain upon physical exertion or emotional stress is characteristic of _____.

2. Atherosclerosis is due to a buildup of fatty, fibrous material called _____ in the walls of arteries.

3. The type of angina pectoris that is predictable in its frequency and duration is called _____ angina.

4. Drug therapy of stable angina usually begins with _____.

5. Long-acting nitrates are often delivered through a _____ to decrease the frequency and severity of anginal episodes.

6. A myocardial infarction is the result of a sudden occlusion of a _____.

7. After a clot in the coronary artery has been successfully dissolved, therapy with _____ is often initiated to prevent the formation of additional thrombi.

8. Stroke is caused by either a _____ or _____ within a vessel serving the brain.

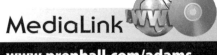

MediaLink

www.prenhall.com/adams

CD-ROM
Animation:
    Mechanism in Action: Reteplase
    (Retevase)
Audio Glossary
NCLEX Review

Companion Website
NCLEX Review
Dosage Calculations
Case Study
Care Plans
Expanded Key Concepts

9. Drug therapy for thrombotic stroke focuses on two main goals: _____ and _____.

10. When a person has significant coronary artery obstruction, the two most common interventions are _____ and _____.

MATCHING

For questions 11 through 17, match the drug in column I with its classification in column II.

Column I	Column II
11. _____ Diltiazem (Cardizem)	a. Organic nitrate
12. _____ Isosorbide dinitrate (Isordil)	b. Beta-blocker
13. _____ Metoprolol (Lopressor)	c. Calcium channel blocker
14. _____ Atenolol (Tenormin)	d. ACE inhibitor
15. _____ Nifedipine (Procardia)	e. Analgesic
16. _____ Nitroglycerin (Nitrostat)	
17. _____ Amlodipine (Norvasc)	

MULTIPLE CHOICE

18. Which of the following drug classes is widely used in the pharmacotherapy of angina pectoris?

    a. Calcium channel blockers

    b. ACE inhibitors

    c. HMG-CoA reductase inhibitors

    d. Cardiac glycosides

19. Which of the following best explains the mechanism by which organic nitrates terminate variant angina?

    a. Direct vasodilation of coronary arteries

    b. Slowing heart rate

    c. Stronger force of myocardial contraction

    d. Dilation of peripheral veins, reducing preload

20. What is the condition of having a reduced blood supply to myocardial cells called?

    a. Myocardial infarction

    b. Angina pectoris

    c. Myocardial ischemia

    d. Stroke

21. In assessing a patient with chest pain, the nurse knows that angina is most often preceded by which of the following?

    a. An aura

    b. Physical exertion or emotional excitement

    c. A sensation that the heart has skipped a beat

    d. Severe pain down the left arm

22. The pharmacologic goals for the treatment of angina are usually achieved by which of the following?

    a. Reducing cardiac workload

    b. Increasing heart rate

    c. Increasing force of myocardial contraction

    d. Increasing amount of blood entering the heart

23. By causing venodilation, nitrates reduce the amount of blood returning to the heart, thus decreasing which of the following?

    a. Heart rate

    b. Conduction velocity

    c. Ischemia

    d. Cardiac output

24. In addition to causing venodilation, organic nitrates have what other ability?

    a. Inhibit alpha$_1$-adrenergic receptors in arterioles

    b. Dilate the coronary arteries

    c. Terminate dysrhythmias

    d. Remove plaque from coronary arteries

25. Organic nitrates are classified based upon whether they are one or the other of the following:

    a. Parenteral or oral

    b. High or low potency

    c. Short or long acting

    d. Sedating or nonsedating

26. Which drug would the nurse administer sublingually to terminate anginal pain?

    a. Atenolol (Tenormin)

    b. Diltiazem (Cardizem)

    c. Nitroglycerin (Nitro-Bid)

    d. Aspirin (Bayer)

27. The nurse should monitor for the most common side effect of nitroglycerin therapy, which is:

    a. Headache

b. Drowsiness

c. Nausea/vomiting

d. Hypotension

28. What is the primary mechanism by which beta-adrenergic blockers decrease the frequency of angina attacks?

    a. Dilating the coronary arteries

    b. Increasing the heart rate

    c. Increasing the strength of contraction of the myocardium

    d. Reducing cardiac workload

29. Which of the following is true regarding the effect of atenolol (Tenormin) on the heart?

    a. Selectively blocks $beta_1$-receptors

    b. Nonselective $beta_1$-and $beta_2$-blocker

    c. Selectively blocks $beta_2$-receptors

    d. Has no effect on beta-receptors

30. What is the primary mechanism by which calcium channel blockers decrease the frequency of angina attacks?

    a. Slowing conduction through the SA node

    b. Increasing the heart rate

    c. Increasing the strength of contraction of the myocardium

    d. Reducing cardiac workload

31. Calcium channel blockers are useful in treating variant angina because they do which of the following?

    a. Lower blood pressure

    b. Slow the heart rate

    c. Slow conduction across the myocardium

    d. Relax arterial smooth muscle in the coronary arteries

32. Which of the following agents has the ability to inhibit the transport of calcium ions into myocardial cells, and the ability to relax both coronary and peripheral blood vessels?

    a. Atenolol (Tenormin)

    b. Diltiazem (Cardizem)

    c. Nitroglycerin (Nitro-Bid)

    d. Reteplase (Retavase)

33. Which of the following is *not* a goal for the pharmacotherapy of acute MI?

    a. Restore blood supply to the damaged myocardium as quickly as possible

    b. Increase myocardial oxygen demand with organic nitrates or beta-blockers

    c. Prevent associated dysrhythmias with antidysrhythmics

    d. Reduce post-MI mortality with aspirin and ACE inhibitors

34. In treating a patient with a recent MI, the nurse knows that the function of thrombolytic therapy is to do which of the following?

    a. Restore blood supply to the damaged myocardium

    b. Decrease myocardial oxygen demand

    c. Control dysrhythmias

    d. Reduce acute pain associated with MI

35. What is the primary risk of thrombolytics?

    a. Hypertension

    b. Prolonged prothrombin time

    c. Excessive bleeding

    d. Dysrhythmia

36. The nurse should know that reteplase (Retavase) is most effective if given within what time frame after the onset of MI symptoms?

    a. 30 minutes

    b. 1 hour

    c. 6 hours

    d. 12 hours

37. Following an acute MI, metoprolol (Lopressor) is infused slowly until which of the following occurs?

    a. The clot is dissolved.

    b. Blood pressure falls to 100/70 mm Hg.

    c. A target heart rate of 60 to 90 beats per minute is reached.

    d. The pain is relieved.

38. Unless contraindicated, 160 to 324 mg of aspirin is given as soon as possible following a suspected MI in order to do which of the following?

    a. Restore blood supply to the damaged myocardium

    b. Decrease myocardial oxygen demand

    c. Reduce post-MI mortality

    d. Reduce acute pain associated with MI

39. Why is captopril (Capoten) sometimes given to MI patients?

    a. To restore blood supply to the damaged myocardium

    b. To increase myocardial oxygen demand

    c. To reduce post-MI mortality

    d. To reduce acute pain associated with MI

40. Why are opioids such as morphine sulfate sometimes given to an MI patient?

    a. To restore blood supply to the damaged myocardium

b. To decrease myocardial oxygen demand

c. To reduce post-MI mortality

d. To reduce acute pain associated with MI

41. Patients at high risk for stroke are often treated with which of the following?

a. Antidysrhythmics

b. Antihypertensives

c. Opioids

d. Cardiac glycosides

MAKING CONNECTIONS

42. In addition to angina, the nurse may administer organic nitrates to treat which of the following?

a. Dysrhythmias

b. Coagulation disorders

c. Hypertension

d. Heart failure

43. What is the classification of nitrous oxide?

a. IV anesthetic

b. Gas

c. Volatile agent

d. Local anesthetic

44. The nurse must ensure that protamine sulfate is available to treat possible excessive bleeding due to which of the following?

a. Hemophilia

b. Heparin overdose

c. Warfarin overdose

d. Deficiency of vitamin K

45. The antidysrhythmic action of lidocaine (Xylocaine) is due to blockade of which of the following?

a. Sodium channels

b. Calcium channels

c. Beta-adrenergic receptors

d. Potassium channels

46. Which of the following blocks impulses from the parasympathetic nervous system?

a. Sympathomimetic

b. Beta-adrenergic blocker

c. Cholinergic blocker

d. Calcium channel blocker

CALCULATIONS

47. A nitroglycerin solution of 50 mg/250 ml D5W is infused at 15 gtt/min. The IV set calibration is 60 gtt/ml. How many mcg/min are infused?

48. A patient has an IV drip of Cardizem 125 mg/100 ml D5W. The doctor orders Cardizem 10 mg/hr. How many drops per minute will the nurse give if a microdrip is used?

CASE STUDY APPLICATIONS

49. Mr. M is a 70-year-old, 280-pound patient admitted through the emergency room for a possible stroke. His physical exam reveals he is alert, with a pulse of 76 regular, BP 190/110 mm Hg, respirations 24/min, and slurred speech. He has significant weakness in the left arm, left hand, and left leg. CT scan confirms a recent CVA. His social history includes occasional alcohol use and two packs per day tobacco use for 50 years. He is a retired accountant, is married, and has seven adult children and 16 grandchildren. During hospitalization, he was given reteplase (Retavase), furosemide (Lasix), and heparin. He was discharged with the following medications: hydrochlorothiazide (HydroDIURIL), diltiazem (Cardizem), and warfarin (Coumadin).

    a. After analysis of the admission data, what risk factors have likely contributed to this patient's stroke?

    b. What presenting symptoms help the nurse to confirm the diagnosis of stroke?

    c. After you review the medications, what rationale supports the delivery of Retavase, Lasix, and heparin?

    d. You are preparing to begin discharge teaching. What rationale will you give Mr. M for the use of hydrochlorothiazide, warfarin, and diltiazem?

50. Mrs. R is a 72-year-old patient who has been treated several times for chronic heart failure, hypertension, and angina. Her current complaint is the frequency and intensity of her anginal pain. She has chest pain with minor exertion and headaches with the use of PRN nitroglycerin. Her current medications are isosorbide dinitrate, nitroglycerin, atenolol, and amlodipine. Physical exam reveals patient is alert, oriented, BP 164/92 mm Hg, pulse 66 regular, respirations 28, skin cool, strength equal in all extremities, edema in lower extremities, weight gain of 7 pounds in 3 weeks.

    a. After analysis of this patient situation, what nursing diagnoses can you identify?

    b. What assessment data support the possibility of side effects from Norvasc?

    c. Why do you think the nitrates are not relieving Mrs. R's pain?

CHAPTER 26

DRUGS FOR SHOCK

OBJECTIVES

To view the objectives, please refer to the textbook, student CD-ROM, and the Companion Website at *www.prenhall.com/adams*.

FILL IN THE BLANK

From the textbook, find the correct word(s) to complete the statement(s).

1. Shock is a clinical syndrome characterized by collapse of the

   _____ system.

2. In the early stages of shock, the body compensates for the fall

   in blood pressure by increasing the activity of the _____ nervous system.

3. Norepinephrine (Levarterenol) acts directly on _____-adrenergic receptors to raise blood pressure.

4. Dopamine selectively stimulates _____-receptors, whereas at higher doses it stimulates

   _____-receptors.

5. Dopamine is used to increase the force of the myocardial contraction by stimulating _____-receptors.

6. The first goal in the treatment of shock is to provide _____.

7. _____ is indicated for the treatment of acute, massive blood loss.

8. The major adverse outcome when using a colloid to treat shock is _____.

9. Signs and symptoms of an allergic response include _____, _____, _____,

   and _____.

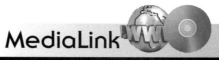

MediaLink

www.prenhall.com/adams

CD-ROM
Animation:
   Mechanism in Action: Dopamine
Audio Glossary
NCLEX Review

Companion Website
NCLEX Review
Dosage Calculations
Case Study
Care Plans
Expanded Key Concepts

10. When given in large doses, hetastarch can increase _____, _____, and

_____.

MATCHING

For questions 11 through 18, match the drug in column I with its primary class in column II.

Column I	Column II
11. Norepinephrine (Levarterenol)	a. Vasoconstrictor
12. Digoxin (Lanoxin)	b. Inotropic
13. Diphenhydramine (Benadryl)	c. Other
14. Mephentermine (Wyamine)	
15. Dopamine (Dopastat)	
16. Albuterol (Proventil)	
17. Methoxamine (Vasoxyl)	
18. Dobutamine (Dobutrex)	

MULTIPLE CHOICE

19. Which of the following would most likely occur in a patient experiencing an overdose of epinephrine?

    a. Hypoglycemia

    b. Hypertension

    c. Bronchospasm

    d. Diarrhea

20. Shock is a condition characterized by which of the following?

    a. Extremely high blood pressure

    b. Abnormal cardiac rhythm

    c. Vital tissues not receiving enough blood to function properly

    d. The heart not pumping with sufficient contractility

21. Which of the following is *not* a common sign or symptom of shock?

    a. Feeling weak, with no specific symptoms

    b. Restlessness, anxiety, confusion, lack of interest

    c. Thirst

    d. Hypertension

22. A weak or unresponsive patient with obvious trauma or bleeding to a limb might be experiencing what type of shock?

    a. Hypovolemic

    b. Neurogenic

    c. Cardiogenic

    d. Anaphylactic

23. In many types of shock, what is the most serious medical challenge facing the patient?

    a. Heart failure

    b. Brain damage

    c. Hypotension

    d. MI

24. What is the purpose of administering vasoconstrictors to a patient with shock?

    a. To prevent dysrhythmias

    b. To stabilize blood pressure

    c. To prevent post shock mortality

    d. To prevent blood pressure from rising to harmful levels

25. Most of the agents used to raise blood pressure in patients with shock:

    a. Are CNS stimulants

    b. Are CNS depressants

    c. Activate the parasympathetic nervous system

    d. Activate the sympathetic nervous system

26. Norepinephrine (Levarterenol) activates which adrenergic receptors?

    a. Alpha

    b. $Beta_1$

    c. Both alpha and $beta_1$

    d. Neither alpha nor $beta_1$

27. In addition to its use in shock, norepinephrine is also of value in treating which of the following?

    a. Cardiac arrest

    b. Hypertension

    c. Dysrhythmias

    d. Strokes

28. The primary use of cardiotonic drugs in the treatment of shock is to increase which of the following?

    a. Blood pressure

    b. Force of myocardial contraction

    c. Heart rate

    d. Conduction velocity across the myocardium

29. Dobutamine (Dobutrex) is a _____ that has value in the treatment of certain types of shock due to its ability to cause the heart to beat more forcefully, without causing major effects on heart rate.

    a. Selective $beta_1$-blocker

    b. Cholinergic blocker

    c. Cardiac glycoside

    d. $Beta_1$-adrenergic agonist

30. A widespread inflammatory response to bacterial, fungal, or parasitic infection can result in which type of shock?

    a. Cardiogenic

    b. Hypovolemic

    c. Neurogenic

    d. Septic

MAKING CONNECTIONS

31. Which of the following is an expected effect of beta-adrenergic blockers?

    a. Increased heart rate

    b. Lowered blood pressure

    c. Dilation of bronchial smooth muscle

    d. Increased myocardial contractility

32. Which of the following is a cholinergic blocker?

    a. Metoprolol (Lopressor)

    b. Succinylcholine (Anectine)

    c. Neostigmine (Prostigmin)

    d. Atropine sulfate

33. Which of the following is *not* classified as an NSAID?

    a. Acetaminophen

    b. Aspirin

    c. Celecoxib (Celebrex)

    d. Ibuprofen

34. Antiplatelet agents are primarily prescribed to do which of the following?

    a. Lower blood cholesterol

    b. Dissolve thrombi

    c. Prevent thromboembolic disease

    d. Prevent migraines

35. Most barbiturate use in children is limited to which of the following?

    a. Sleep disorders

    b. Seizure disorders

    c. Depression

    d. Anxiety

CALCULATIONS

36. Dopamine has been ordered at 4 mcg/kg/min using a 400 mg/250 ml D5W solution. The patient weighs 92.4 kg. Calculate the dosage per minute and ml/hr flow rate.

37. Dobutrex 5 mcg/kg/min has been ordered using a 500 mg/250 ml D5W solution. The patient weighs 99.4 kg. Calculate the ml/hr flow rate.

CASE STUDY APPLICATIONS

38. Paramedics arrive at the scene of an automobile accident and discover a 35-year-old victim who is wandering around the scene confused. The patient has several superficial wounds that are bleeding, although the amount of blood does not appear to be great. Initial vital signs show slightly elevated blood pressure and weak pulse. The paramedics treat the wounds, administer oxygen, and keep the patient warm and lying on a stretcher while they treat other injured people at the scene. Twenty minutes later, the patient is unresponsive with a blood pressure of 70/40 and no identifiable pulse. EKG reveals a ventricular dysrhythmia that appears to be quickly worsening. The paramedics immediately administer the following drugs:

    dextran 70 (Macrodex)

    norepinephrine (Levophed)

    dobutamine (Dobutrex)

    lidocaine (Xylocaine)

    a. What assessment data support a diagnosis of hypovolemic shock?

    b. What nursing diagnosis would be most appropriate at the scene of this accident?

    c. What is the rationale for each drug and how will you evaluate effectiveness?

39. At the same auto accident described in the previous question, paramedics find an elderly patient who has a closed head injury. The patient is unconscious and has no bleeding evident. Vital signs show slow respirations, very low pulse rate, and a blood pressure of 94/52. Pupils are unresponsive to light.

    a. What type of shock is this patient most likely experiencing? List all assessment data that lead you to this conclusion.

    b. What drugs would you expect to implement to reverse the symptoms of shock?

    c. What data would lead you to evaluate this case as being a successfully treated case of neurogenic shock?

CHAPTER 27

DRUGS FOR LIPID DISORDERS

OBJECTIVES

To view the objectives, please refer to the textbook, student CD-ROM, and the Companion Website at *www.prenhall.com/adams*.

FILL IN THE BLANK

From the textbook, find the correct word(s) to complete the statement(s).

1. The general term that means high levels of lipids in the blood is

   _____.

2. Cholesterol contributes to the fatty _____ that narrows arteries.

3. The three basic types of lipids are _____, _____, and _____.

4. Lipoproteins consist of various amounts of _____, _____, and _____ plus a protein carrier.

5. The _____ class of antihyperlipidemics interferes with a critical enzyme in the synthesis of cholesterol.

6. A male patient having an LDL to HDL ratio greater than _____ is at risk for cardiovascular disease.

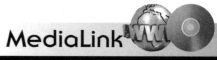

MediaLink

www.prenhall.com/adams

CD-ROM
Animation:
  Mechanism in Action: Atorvastatin
Audio Glossary
NCLEX Review

Companion Website
NCLEX Review
Dosage Calculations
Case Study
Care Plans
Expanded Key Concepts

MATCHING

For questions 7 through 10, match the drug in column I with its primary class in column II.

Column I	Column II
7. _____ Cholestyramine (Questran)	a. HMG-CoA reductase inhibitor
8. _____ Nicotinic acid	b. Bile acid–binding agent
9. _____ Gemfibrozil (Lopid)	c. Fibric acid agent
10. _____ Atorvastatin (Lipitor)	d. None of the above

MULTIPLE CHOICE

11. Drugs that lower lipids are intended to reduce the likelihood of which of the following?

    a. Dysrhythmias

    b. Colon cancer

    c. Coronary artery disease

    d. Obesity

12. LDL transports cholesterol from the liver to the tissues and organs, where it is used to do which of the following?

    a. Provide energy for cells

    b. Build plasma membranes or to synthesize steroids

    c. Make bile

    d. Make HDL

13. LDL is often called what type of cholesterol, because the lipoprotein contributes significantly to plaque deposits?

    a. Good

    b. Bad

    c. High

    d. Low

14. What happens to the cholesterol component of HDL after it is transported to the liver?

    a. It is used to make LDL.

    b. It is used to build plasma membranes.

    c. It is used as an energy source.

    d. It is broken down to become part of bile.

15. Which of the following is *not* a lifestyle change that should be considered by patients with high blood lipid levels?

    a. Maintain weight at an optimum level

    b. Implement a medically supervised exercise plan

    c. Reduce sources of stress

    d. Limit soluble fiber in the diet to 2 or fewer grams per day

16. Which of the following should be monitored carefully during the first few months of therapy with statins?

    a. Blood pressure

    b. Sleep patterns

    c. Cardiac function

    d. Liver function

17. Bile acid resins act by doing which of the following?

    a. Inhibiting HMG-CoA reductase

    b. Increasing excretion of cholesterol in the feces

    c. Decreasing production of HDL

    d. Decreasing absorption of dietary lipids

18. Which of the following is *not* true regarding cholestyramine (Questran)?

    a. It is not absorbed or metabolized once it enters the intestine.

    b. It acts by inhibiting cholesterol biosynthesis.

    c. Its most frequent side effects are constipation, bloating, gas, and nausea.

    d. It should not be taken at the same time as other medications.

19. Which of the following is a B-complex vitamin?

    a. Nicotinic acid

    b. Gemfibrozil (Lopid)

    c. Lovastatin (Mevacor)

    d. Colestipol (Colestid)

20. Which of the following best describes the use of nicotinic acid in treating hyperlipidemias?

    a. It should never be used in patients with hypercholesterolemia.

    b. It should never be used in patients with a history of heart failure.

    c. It should never be used with other antilipidemics, because their effects may cancel each other.

    d. It is most often used in lower doses in combination with a statin.

21. Which of the following should be taken separately from other medications, because it may interfere with drug absorption?

    a. Nicotinic acid

    b. Gemfibrozil (Lopid)

    c. Cholestyramine (Questran)

    d. Fluvastatin (Lescol)

MAKING CONNECTIONS

22. Which of the following best describes propranolol (Inderal)?

    a. Central-acting antihypertensive

    b. Beta-adrenergic blocker

    c. Glycoprotein IIb/IIIa inhibitor

    d. Nonnarcotic analgesic

23. Which of the following is *not* a therapeutic effect of aspirin?

    a. Increase PT time

    b. Prevent heart attack

    c. Relief of severe pain

    d. Reduction of inflammation

24. You are giving simvastatin (Zocor) to all of the following patients. Which patient diagnosis causes you to question the delivery of Zocor?

    a. Atrial fibrillation with warfarin treatment

    b. Osteoporosis with calcium supplement

    c. Hypertension with Lasix treatment

    d. Asthma with Alupent updraft

25. Which of the following is true regarding category D drugs?

    a. They may be safely used in pregnant patients.

    b. Animal studies indicate some risk, but the drug appears to be safe for humans.

    c. They should only be used in pregnant patients if the potential benefit justifies the potential risk to the fetus.

    d. They should not be used in pregnant patients under any circumstance.

26. Which of the following is used to treat seizures?

    a. Thiopental sodium (Pentothal)

    b. Fluoxetine (Prozac)

    c. Valproic acid (Depakote)

    d. Haloperidol (Haldol)

CALCULATIONS

27. The physician orders simvastatin (Zocor) 40 mg qhs. The supply is 40 mg tablets scored. How many tablets will the nurse give the patient, and at what time?

28. The nurse practitioner orders gemfibrozil (Lopid) 1.2 g daily in two divided doses. The pharmacy sends several 600 mg scored tablets. How many tablets will the nurse give, and at what time?

CASE STUDY APPLICATIONS

29. Mr. S is a 57-year-old obese patient who has a history of two heart attacks over the past 3 years. He has been treated with antihypertensives for a 3-year history of hypertension. LDL cholesterol was recently measured at 190 mg/dl and triglycerides were 900 mg/dl. The patient does not smoke, and walks 0.25 mile twice a week.

    a. What data can you identify from the initial assessment that would support a nursing diagnosis of Deficit knowledge: Disease process and lifestyle implications of coronary heart disease?

    b. Does the clinical history warrant the implementation of antihyperlipidemic therapy? Why?

    c. As you evaluate this patient's history, what lifestyle suggestions might you offer?

30. Ms. G is a 35-year-old patient who is 25 pounds overweight. She exercises regularly and has been taking 40 mg/day of atorvastatin (Lipitor) for the past 2 years. Although her blood lipid profile was normal 12 months ago, her lipid levels have slowly risen to 1000 mg/dl (normal 400 to 800 mg/dl).

    a. How do you evaluate this change in lipid level?

    b. What teaching plan would you implement to help these lipid levels return to normal?

CHAPTER 28

DRUGS FOR HEMATOPOIETIC DISORDERS

OBJECTIVES

To view the objectives, please refer to the textbook, student CD-ROM, and the Companion Website at *www.prenhall.com/adams*.

FILL IN THE BLANK

From the textbook, find the correct word(s) to complete the statement(s).

1. Blood serves all body cells and is the only _____ tissue.

2. Over _____ new blood cells are formed every day.

3. Red blood cell formation, also known as _____, is regulated by the hormone _____.

4. Human erythropoietin is marketed as the drug _____.

5. Production of white blood cells is more complicated than erythropoiesis because of the many

   _____ of _____ in the blood.

6. A single megakaryocyte can produce thousands of _____.

7. Classification of anemia is generally based on the _____ and _____ of the erythrocyte.

8. _____ and _____ maintain iron stores inside cells.

9. _____ transports iron to sites in the body where it is needed.

10. After erythrocytes die, most of the iron in their hemoglobin is _____ for later use.

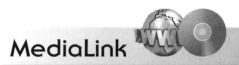

MediaLink

www.prenhall.com/adams

CD-ROM
Audio Glossary
NCLEX Review

Companion Website
NCLEX Review
Dosage Calculations
Case Study
Care Plans
Expanded Key Concepts

MATCHING

For questions 11 through 18, match the indication in column I with its drug in column II.

	Column I	Column II
11. _____	Pernicious anemia	a. Epoetin alfa
12. _____	Anemic HIV-infected patient	b. Filgrastim
13. _____	AIDS-related immunosuppression	c. Cyanocobalamin
14. _____	Anemia caused by chemotherapy	d. Ferrous sulfate
15. _____	Neutropenia caused by chemotherapy	
16. _____	Chronic renal failure	
17. _____	Megaloblastic anemia	
18. _____	Anemia from peptic ulcer disease	

MULTIPLE CHOICE

19. Nursing interventions for patients receiving hematopoietic growth factor therapy include all *except* which of the following?

    a. Assess for a history of uncontrolled hypertension

    b. Assess for food or drug allergies

    c. Assess for signs of liver dysfunction

    d. Monitor patient for early signs of CVA or MI

20. Examples of colony-stimulating factors improving the function of cells include all *except* which of the following?

    a. Increased migration of leukocytes to antigens

    b. Increased antibody toxicity

    c. Rapid platelet production

    d. Increased phagocytosis

21. Patients who are neutropenic secondary to chemotherapy treatments can be expected to receive which of the following?

    a. Erythropoietin

    b. Filgrastim

    c. Oprelvekin

    d. Sargramostim

22. Your patient is receiving an IV infusion of sargramostim. He develops dyspnea, rapid pulse, hypotension, and complains of feeling dizzy. What should you do?

    a. Telephone the doctor STAT and prepare to administer epinephrine.

    b. Assess the patient for an allergy to yeast.

    c. Check a CBC and differential.

    d. Discontinue the IV, then restart it at half the previous rate after the symptoms are gone.

23. Patient teaching for filgrastim includes all *except* which of the following?

    a. Take medication with a full glass of water to decrease the risk of kidney damage.

    b. Wash hands frequently and avoid people with infections.

    c. Report chest pain, palpitations, respiratory problems, fever, chills, and malaise to the doctor immediately.

    d. Keep all laboratory and doctor appointments.

24. What is the only suitable route when administering oprelvekin?

    a. PO

    b. IV

    c. SC

    d. IM

25. Which of the following statements about vitamin B_{12} is false?

    a. It can be synthesized by certain plants.

    b. It can be synthesized by bacteria.

    c. Very small amounts of B_{12} are required daily.

    d. The most common cause of B_{12} deficiency is lack of the intrinsic factor.

26. Which of the following statements about pernicious anemia is false?

    a. It affects more than one body system.

    b. The stem cells produce abnormally large leukocytes that do not fully mature.

    c. Permanent nervous system damage may result if the disease remains untreated.

    d. Intrinsic factor is required to prevent the disease.

27. Which of the following is *not* a common cause of iron deficiency?

    a. Blood loss

    b. Pregnancy

    c. Intensive athletic training

    d. Kidney disease

28. Which of these statements regarding iron preparations is false?

    a. Prior to administering an IV dose, the patient must receive a test dose.

    b. Iron should be taken with food to increase absorption.

    c. Iron may cause nausea, vomiting, and constipation.

    d. Iron may turn stools dark green or black.

29. Which of the following drugs must be given using the Z-track method?

    a. Iron dextran

    b. Cyanocobalamin

    c. Filgrastim

    d. Epoetin alfa

30. Which of the following statements regarding folic acid is false?

    a. It does not require intrinsic factor for intestinal absorption.

    b. The most common cause is insufficient dietary intake.

    c. Deficiency is commonly seen in chronic alcoholics.

    d. It is unsafe to take this preparation during pregnancy.

MAKING CONNECTIONS

31. An anticholinergic drug is one that blocks the effects of which of the following?

    a. Epinephrine

    b. Norepinephrine

    c. Acetylcholine

    d. Serotonin

32. Which major depolarizing neuromuscular blocker used during surgery?

    a. Succinylcholine (Anectine)

    b. Acetylcholine

    c. Promethazine (Phenergan)

    d. Bethanechol (Urecholine)

33. Which of the following would be used to treat mild to moderate pain due to inflammation?

    a. Oxycodone (OxyContin)

    b. Meperidine (Demerol)

    c. Ibuprofen (Advil)

    d. Acetaminophen (Tylenol)

34. What antagonist may be administered if serious hemorrhage occurs during heparin therapy?

    a. Protamine sulfate

    b. Vitamin K

    c. Adenosine diphosphate (ADP)

    d. Desmopressin (DDAVP)

35. Which of the following would be used to lower extremely high blood pressure within minutes?

    a. Hydralazine (Apresoline)

    b. Nitroprusside (Nitropress)

    c. Doxazosin (Cardura)

    d. Prazosin (Minipress)

CALCULATIONS

36. How much filgrastim would the nurse give a patient who weighs 57 kg, for whom the minimum dose of 5 mcg/kg/day is ordered subcutaneously?

37. A pediatric patient weighs 66 pounds. The physician has ordered a subcutaneous daily dose of filgrastim 750 mcg. The maximum recommended SQ dose is 20/mcg/kg/day. Is this dose within the recommended limits?

CASE STUDY APPLICATIONS

38. Mr. B is a 58-year-old patient who is coming to the dialysis clinic three times a week. He is receiving Epogen injections after each treatment.

    a. What information can you give this patient regarding why he needs to receive erythropoietin?

    b. What side effects of erythropoietin should be assessed during each clinic visit?

    c. Since one of your goals for this patient is "to promote patient independence regarding self-care", what patient education is necessary for Mr. B?

39. Mr. J, age 63, has been admitted to your unit with a diagnosis of megaloblastic anemia. He complains of feeling tired and weak. He states, "I just can't make myself do anything." Mr. J has a history of gout and chronic gastritis. He wants to know why he is not on an iron preparation, since that is how a friend's anemia was treated. Further assessment reveals that Mr. J has virtually no knowledge of his disease or treatment. Your nursing care plan includes teaching interventions to address this knowledge deficit.

    a. You are evaluating Mr. J's understanding of why he feels tired and weak. What should he tell you?

    b. What information would you give Mr. J regarding self-care?

    c. How would you explain to Mr. J that an iron preparation is probably not the answer to his problem?

40. Mrs. Z has been receiving chemotherapy for her cancer. She is admitted to your unit with a diagnosis of neutropenia. She has been started on filgrastim injections and placed on neutropenic precautions.

    a. What assessments must you make prior to giving Mrs. Z her first injection of filgrastim?

    b. What information would you give this patient regarding side effects of her medication?

    c. While evaluating Mrs. Z's understanding of your teaching, you ask her to tell you how she can decrease her risk of getting an infection. What should she be able to tell you?

CHAPTER 29

DRUGS FOR PULMONARY DISORDERS

OBJECTIVES

To view the objectives, please refer to the textbook, student CD-ROM, and the Companion Website at *www.prenhall.com/adams*.

FILL IN THE BLANK

From the text book, find the correct word(s) to complete the statement(s).

1. The two main physiologic processes of the respiratory system

   are _____ and _____.

2. A machine that vaporizes a liquid drug into a fine mist that

   can be inhaled is called a _____.

3. The two primary disorders classified as COPDs are

   _____ and _____.

4. The process of gas exchange is called _____.

5. The respiratory rate, which is normally _____ per minute, can be modified by factors such as

   _____, _____, _____, and _____.

6. Stimulation of the parasympathetic nervous system results in bronchiole _____.

7. _____ uses a propellant to deliver a measured dose of drug to the lung during each breath.

8. _____ is a severe, prolonged form of asthma that is unresponsive to drug therapy and may lead to respiratory failure.

9. Goals of drug therapy for asthma are twofold: to _____ acute bronchospasm and to reduce the

   _____ of asthma attacks.

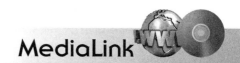

10. The most commonly used nonnarcotic antitussive is _____.

MATCHING

For questions 11 through 19, match the drug in column I with its primary class in column II.

Column I	Column II
11. _____ Triamcinolone (Azmacort)	a. Selective beta$_2$-agonist
12. _____ Epinephrine (Adrenalin, Bronkaid, Primatene)	b. Nonselective beta$_1$-and beta$_2$-agonist
13. _____ Albuterol (Proventil, Salbutamol, others)	c. Methylxanthine
14. _____ Isoproterenol (Isuprel, Medihaler-Iso)	d. Anticholinergic
15. _____ Budesonide (Pulmicort Turbuhaler)	e. Glucocorticoid
16. _____ Salmeterol (Serevent)	
17. _____ Ipratropium (Atrovent, Combivent)	
18. _____ Aminophylline (Truphylline)	
19. _____ Fluticasone (Flovent)	

For questions 20 through 24, match the description in column I with its drug in column II.

Column I	Column II
20. A natural therapy purported to restore normal secretions to lung and other organs	a. Benzonatate (Tessalon)
21. A medication used to directly loosen thick, viscous bronchial secretions	b. Guaifenesin
22. Most effective over-the-counter expectorant	c. Dextromethorphan
23. Nonopiate antitussive having few side effects	d. Acetylcysteine (Mucomyst)
24. Nonopiate that acts by anesthetizing stretch receptors in the lung	e. Horehound

MULTIPLE CHOICE

25. During inspiration, air leaving the trachea next enters which area of the body?

    a. Pharynx

    b. Bronchioles

    c. Alveoli

    d. Bronchi

26. Exchange of gasses occurs in which pulmonary structure?

    a. Pharynx

    b. Bronchioles

    c. Alveoli

    d. Bronchi

27. When assessing a patient, the nurse must know that which of the following is *not* characteristic of asthma?

    a. Inflammation

    b. Infection

    c. Bronchoconstriction

    d. Dyspnea

28. Which of the following classes would *least* likely be prescribed for asthma?

    a. Beta$_2$-agonists

    b. Methylxanthines

    c. Glucocorticoids

    d. Beta-blockers

29. Which of the following drug classes is *most* effective for relieving acute bronchospasm?

    a. Beta$_2$-agonists

    b. Mast cell stabilizers

    c. Methylxanthines

    d. Anticholinergics

30. The nurse should teach the patient that salmeterol (Serevent) is *not* indicated for the termination of acute bronchospasm for which of the following reasons?

    a. It is not absorbed orally.

    b. It takes too long to act.

    c. It affects only beta$_1$-receptors.

    d. It causes too much CNS stimulation.

31. When administering glucocorticoids for the prophylaxis of nonpersistent asthma, the nurse should know that these drugs are most commonly administered by which route?

    a. Oral

    b. Topical

    c. Intranasal

    d. Intradermal

32. Glucocorticoids improve asthma symptoms by which of the following mechanisms?

    a. Causing bronchodilation

    b. Suppressing inflammation

    c. Blocking histamine release

    d. Drying bronchial secretions

33. The nurse should teach the patient that long-term treatment with oral corticosteroids may cause which serious adverse effect?

    a. Rebound congestion

    b. Hypertension

    c. Cancer

    d. Adrenal atrophy

34. The nurse should know that candidiasis of the throat is a common complication during therapy with which class of medications?

    a. Inhaled glucocorticoids

    b. Mast cell stabilizers

    c. Beta$_2$-agonists

    d. Mucolytics

35. The nurse should teach patients that the primary use of mast cell inhibitors in the treatment of asthma is which of the following?

    a. To terminate acute asthmatic attacks

    b. To prevent asthmatic attacks

    c. To reduce secretions

    d. To reduce infections

36. Nedocromil (Tilade) and cromolyn act by which of the following mechanisms?

    a. Causing bronchodilation

    b. Suppressing the cough reflex

    c. Blocking histamine release

    d. Drying bronchial secretions

37. What is the primary action of an antitussive?

    a. Suppress the cough reflex

    b. Dry bronchial secretions

    c. Block histamine release

    d. Reduce the viscosity of bronchial secretions

38. What is the primary action of an expectorant?

    a. Suppress the cough reflex

    b. Dry bronchial secretions

    c. Reduce inflammation

    d. Reduce the viscosity of bronchial secretions

39. The most effective antitussives are from which drug class?

    a. Opioids

    b. Glucocorticoids

  c. Beta$_2$-agonists

  d. NSAIDs

40. Patients taking zafirlukast (Accolate) or montelukast (Singulair) should be taught that they will see improvement within what time frame?

  a. 2 hours

  b. 2 days

  c. 1 week

  d. 1 month

41. What is the most common reason for school absenteeism?

  a. Asthma

  b. Ear infections

  c. Colds

  d. Heart disease

42. Why are selective beta$_1$-agonists ineffective for treating asthma?

  a. There are no beta$_1$-receptors in bronchial smooth muscle.

  b. They cannot be delivered by the inhalation route.

  c. They cause bronchoconstriction.

  d. Their duration of action is too short.

MAKING CONNECTIONS

43. Trizivir is a combination drug that contains abacavir, lamivudine, and zidovudine. This drug is most likely used to treat which infection?

  a. Bacterial

  b. Fungal

  c. Herpes

  d. HIV/AIDS

44. The nurse would administer which of the following for opioid overdose?

  a. Methadone (Dolophine)

  b. Epinephrine (Adrenalin)

  c. Naloxone (Narcan)

  d. Dobutamine (Dobutrex)

45. Which of the following drugs has analgesic, anti-inflammatory, and antipyretic activity?

    a. Morphine sulfate

    b. Aspirin

    c. Acetaminophen

    d. Vicodin (hydrocodone with acetaminophen)

46. Why has the use of penicillin G declined over the past decade?

    a. There are less expensive alternatives.

    b. More people are becoming allergic to the drug.

    c. Other antibiotics are available that cause fewer side effects.

    d. Widespread microbial resistance has developed.

CALCULATIONS

47. A patient has aminophylline ordered at 0.25 mg/kg/hr. The patient weighs 50 kg. How many milligrams should be administered over a 6 hour period?

48. A patient has albuterol 4 mg ordered tid. Concentrate of 2 mg in 5 cc is available. How many milliliters would be given per each dose?

CASE STUDY APPLICATIONS

49. Mr. H has been admitted to a respiratory floor after being treated in the ER for an exacerbation of asthma. The patient states he has been on beclomethasone (Beconase) inhaler and an oral theophylline preparation for about 2 months. His last exacerbation of asthma was about 2 months ago, and he claims to be compliant with his medications. About a week ago, Mr. H started having a persistent cough, productive of green thick sputum. He has been short of breath and has been wheezing in the ER. The physician prescribes lorazepam (Ativan) and metaproterenol (Alupent) while Mr. H is in the ER. The nurse has chosen a nursing diagnosis of ineffective airway clearance due to infective process causing increased mucous production.

    a. Which assessment would indicate a possible infection and ineffective airway clearance?

    b. Which nursing interventions would need to be completed for the diagnosis of ineffective airway clearance?

    c. Give the therapeutic rationales for the two drugs taken by Mr. H prior to the ER visit.

    d. Give the therapeutic rationales for the two drugs taken by Mr. H during his ER visit.

50. Ms. D comes to a clinic with history of a cold. She has been self-medicating with acetaminophen (Tylenol), diphenhydramine (Benadryl), and pseudoephedrine (Sudafed). The patient now presents with an earache and a nonproductive cough and wheezing. The physician provides the patient with a prescription for Robitussin AC and a Proventil inhaler. He tells Ms. D to continue to take pseudoephedrine and acetaminophen. He also prescribes an antibiotic for her ear infection. The patient asks you why she can't take diphenhydramine and why the doctor's choice of medications would be better than hers.

    a. What nursing diagnosis would you choose for the patient?

    b. Which interventions would you need to complete for the patient?

CHAPTER 30

DRUGS FOR IMMUNE SYSTEM MODULATION

OBJECTIVES

To view the objectives, please refer to the textbook, student CD-ROM, and the Companion Website at *www.prenhall.com/adams*.

FILL IN THE BLANK

From the textbook, find the correct word(s) to complete the statement(s).

1. Foreign agents that elicit an immune response are referred to

    as _____.

2. The body's second line of defense that is specific against certain pathogens is referred to as the

    _____.

3. B cells initiate _____ immunity and secrete _____ that neutralize or mark the antigen for destruction by other cells in the immune system.

4. When the patient's immune system is stimulated to produce antibodies due to exposure to a specific antigen, it is referred to as _____ immunity.

5. The administration of gamma globulin after the exposure to hepatitis is referred to as _____ immunity.

6. _____ is a life-threatening disease that is considered eradicated from the world through immunization.

7. Activated T cells recognize specific antigens and produce hormone-like proteins called _____ that regulate the intensity and duration of the immune response.

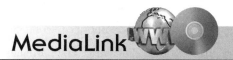

8. Immunostimulants, referred to as _____, have been approved to boost certain functions of the immune system.

9. Immunosuppressants are effective at inhibiting a patient's immune system, but must be monitored carefully as loss of immune function can lead to _____.

10. Four drug classes used to dampen the immune response are _____, _____, _____, and_____.

MATCHING

For questions 11 through 16, match the drug in column I to the primary class in column II.

Column I	Column II
11. _____ Interferon alfa–2 (Roferon-A, Intron A)	a. Calcineurin inhibitor
12. _____ Cyclosporine (Neoral, Sandimmune)	b. Immune globulin preparation
13. _____ Poliovirus, oral (Orimune)	c. Immunostimulant
14. _____ Rituximab (Rituxan)	d. Vaccine
15. _____ Azathioprine (Imuran)	e. Antibody
16. _____ Cytomegalovirus immune globulin (CytoGam)	f. Antimetabolite/cytotoxic agent

MULTIPLE CHOICE

17. Foreign agents that elicit a specific immune response are referred to as which of the following?
    a. Immunoglobulins
    b. Cytokines
    c. Antigens
    d. Antibodies

18. A nurse must understand the interrelationships in the immune system, and one of those relationships is the primary function of plasma cells to secrete which of the following?
    a. Complement
    b. Histamine
    c. Antibodies
    d. Cytokines

19. Memory B cells are programmed to remember the initial antigen interaction. Should the body be exposed to the same antigen in the future, the body manufactures high levels of antibodies in approximately what time frame?
    a. 2 to 3 hours
    b. 2 to 3 days

c. 2 to 3 weeks

d. 2 to 3 months

20. Which drugs must be administered to avoid the body's rejection of an organ transplant?

a. COX–2 inhibitors

b. H$_2$-receptor antagonists

c. Immunosuppressants

d. Systemic glucocorticoids

21. Which drug produces its therapeutic effects by inhibiting T cells?

a. Cyclosporine (Sandimmune)

b. Prednisone

c. Aspirin

d. Celecoxib (Celebrex)

22. When monitoring a patient for primary adverse effects from cyclosporine, the nurse must be aware that these adverse effects occur in which of the following areas?

a. Immune system

b. Lung

c. GI tract

d. Kidney

23. Which is *not* a type of vaccine suspension?

a. Live microbes

b. Killed microbes

c. Microbes that are alive but attenuated

d. Bacterial toxins

24. To present effective patient education, the nurse must know that the purpose of a vaccine is which of the following?

a. To treat active infections

b. To prevent inflammation, should an infection occur

c. To prevent infections from occurring

d. To suppress the immune system so that hypersensitivity to antigens does not occur

25. During patient education, the nurse needs to understand that a toxoid is classified as which of the following?

a. Vaccine

b. Immunosuppressant

c. Anti-inflammatory agent

d. Antigen

26. Which biologic response modifier would be prescribed for the treatment of Kaposi's sarcoma?

    a. Interleukin–2

    b. Interleukin–11

    c. Interferon alfa

    d. Interferon beta

27. Which biologic response modifier would be prescribed for the treatment of metastatic renal carcinoma?

    a. Interleukin–2

    b. Interleukin–11

    c. Interferon alfa

    d. Interferon beta

28. Which biologic response modifier is reserved for the treatment of severe multiple sclerosis?

    a. Interleukin–2

    b. Interleukin–11

    c. Interferon alfa

    d. Interferon beta

MAKING CONNECTIONS

29. Which drug administration method has the highest potential for severe adverse effects?

    a. PO

    b. IM

    c. IV

    d. SC

30. Which GABA channel is opened by benzodiazepines such as diazepam?

    a. Na^+

    b. K^+

    c. Cl^-

    d. Ca^{+2}

31. For which disorder are neuroleptic drugs used for treatment?

    a. Clinical depression

    b. Bipolar disorder

    c. Psychosis

    d. ADD

32. Which is a potential early adverse effect from nitrous oxide?

    a. Restlessness or anxiety

    b. Dysrhythmia

c. Hypertension

d. Mania

33. Which primary action of digoxin (Lanoxin) is effective in the treatment of heart failure?

    a. It dilates the coronary arteries.

    b. It increases impulse conduction across the myocardium.

    c. It decreases blood pressure.

    d. It increases cardiac contractility/output.

CALCULATIONS

34. Mr. K is to receive cytomegalovirus immune globulin (CytoGam). The order reads: to be given IV 150 mg/kg within 72 hours of transplantation, then 100 mg/kg 2, 4, 6, and 8 wk post transplant, then 50 mg/kg 12 and 16 wk post transplant. Mr. K weighs 180 lb. How many mg will he receive in 72 hours, 2, 4, 6, 8, 12, and 16 wk?

35. Ms. B. is to receive tacrolimus (Prograf) 0.15 mg/kg/day q12h. She weighs 100 lb. How many mg will she receive in 12h and in 24h?

CASE STUDY APPLICATIONS

36. Mrs. L has been diagnosed with hairy cell leukemia and it has been recommended that she begin receiving immunostimulant therapy. During the initial physical assessment it was determined that she is 6 weeks' pregnant. Since the physician has determined that interferon beta–1b is the appropriate drug for this condition, the nurse must carefully monitor the patient for signs of complications related to the drug therapy and status of the pregnancy.

    a. What possible adverse reaction can this drug have on pregnancy?

    b. What complications and/or adverse reactions do immunostimulants cause?

    c. What side effects should patients taking immunostimulants be instructed to report to their primary nurse?

37. Ms. H recently received a kidney transplant and is being released to go home. The nurse discharging her determines that extensive patient education regarding the purpose, action, and possible adverse reactions to immunosuppressants is necessary for the future well-being of this patient.

    a. What is the purpose of immunosuppressants, and for how long will it be necessary for Ms. H to receive this drug therapy?

    b. Explain the action of this class of drugs.

    c. What are the possible adverse reactions to this drug therapy?

38. A.J. is 1-year old and has just received his measles, mumps, and rubella (MMR II). His mother is not sure why her son needs to have "all of these shots." The nurse explains to A. J.'s mother the rationale for her son receiving the vaccinations. The nurse also presents information on the possible adverse reactions, and explains that severe reactions to vaccinations are rare.

    a. What rationale would you give the mother for the vaccinations?

    b. For what adverse reactions would you teach the mother to monitor?

CHAPTER 31

DRUGS FOR INFLAMMATION, FEVER, AND ALLERGIES

OBJECTIVES

To view the objectives, please refer to the textbook, student CD-ROM, and the Companion Website at *www.prenhall.com/adams*.

FILL IN THE BLANK

From the textbook, find the correct word(s) to complete the statement(s).

1. The central purpose of inflammation is _____.

2. The fundamental problem of allergic rhinitis is inflammation of the _____ of the nose, throat, and airway.

3. Drug classes used to prevent allergic rhinitis include _____ , _____, and _____.

4. Because the sympathomimetics only relieve nasal congestion, they are often combined with _____ to control the sneezing and tearing of allergic rhinitis.

5. Oral and intranasal _____ are effective at relieving nasal congestion due to the common cold.

6. _____ cells detect foreign agents or injury and respond by releasing histamine.

7. Large amounts of hydrochloric acid are secreted in the stomach in response to the presence of _____.

8. First-line drugs for the treatment of mild to moderate inflammation are the _____.

9. _____ are natural hormones released by the adrenal cortex that have powerful effects on nearly every cell in the body.

10. During long-term therapy with glucocorticoids, the nurse must be alert for signs of a condition referred to as _____ syndrome.

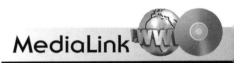

MediaLink

www.prenhall.com/adams

CD-ROM
Animations:
  Mechanism in Action: Diphenhydramine (Benadryl and others)
  Mechanism in Action: Naproxen (Naprosyn)
Audio Glossary
NCLEX Review

Companion Website
NCLEX Review
Dosage Calculations
Case Study
Care Plans
Expanded Key Concepts

MATCHING

For questions 11 through 25, match the primary class in column I with its drug in column II.

<table>
<tr><th>Column I</th><th>Column II</th></tr>
<tr><td>11. _____ Azelastine (Astelin)</td><td>a. H₁-receptor antagonist</td></tr>
</table>

Column I

11. _____ Azelastine (Astelin)

12. _____ Oxymetazoline (Afrin 12 Hour, Neo-Synephrine 12 Hour, others)

13. _____ Dexamethasone (Decadron, others)

14. _____ Fenoprofen (Nalfon)

15. _____ Oxaprozin (Daypro)

16. _____ Mometasone (Nasonex)

17. _____ Diphenhydramine (Benadryl, others)

18. _____ Ephedrine (Primatene)

19. _____ Flunisolide (Nasalide, Nasarel)

20. _____ Prednisolone (Delta-Cortef, Pedi-Cort, others)

21. _____ Celecoxib (Celebrex)

22. _____ Brompheniramine (Dimetapp, others)

23. _____ Clemastine (Tavist)

24. _____ Beclomethasone (Beconase, Vancenase)

25. _____ Pseudoephedrine (Actifed, Sudafed, others)

Column II

a. H$_1$-receptor antagonist

b. Sympathomimetic

c. Intranasal glucocorticoid

d. Nonsteroidal anti-inflammatory drug (NSAID)

e. Systemic (oral) glucocorticoid

MULTIPLE CHOICE

26. The nurse would determine that the use of hydrocortisone would be contraindicated in a patient experiencing which of the following?

   a. An active infection associated with inflammation

   b. Pain associated with inflammation

   c. Nasal congestion

   d. Hypertension

27. What is the primary action of histamine?

   a. Vasodilator

   b. Vasoconstrictor

   c. Sympathomimetic

   d. Cardiotonic agent

28. Rapid release of histamine on a massive scale throughout the body is responsible for which of the following?

    a. Irreversible inhibition of cyclooxygenase

    b. Allergic rhinitis

    c. Immunosuppression

    d. Anaphylaxis

29. The classifications for H_1-receptor antagonists are based on the degree to which the drugs:

    a. Block stomach acid secretion

    b. Affect blood coagulation

    c. Cause xerostomia

    d. Cause drowsiness

30. In the treatment of allergies, why are newer antihistamines an improvement over the older, more traditional antihistamines?

    a. Less sedating

    b. More efficacious

    c. More potent

    d. Less GI irritation

31. Symptoms of motion sickness are often alleviated by treatment with drugs from which class?

    a. H_1-receptor antagonists

    b. H_2-receptor antagonists

    c. Immunosuppressants

    d. Intranasal glucocorticoids

32. Which drug is frequently used in conjunction with analgesics and decongestants?

    a. Fluticasone (Flonase)

    b. Fexofenadine (Allegra)

    c. Diphenhydramine (Benadryl)

    d. Prednisone (Meticorten)

33. Which is the most common adverse effect from therapy with diphenhydramine?

    a. Urinary retention

    b. Dysrhythmia

    c. Drowsiness

    d. Bradycardia

34. Which of the following is the most frequently reported side effect for intranasal glucocorticoids?

    a. Sinus congestion

    b. Tachycardia

    c. Burning sensation in the nose

    d. Dry mouth

35. Which autonomic drug class is commonly used to dry the nasal mucosa?

    a. Sympathomimetics

    b. Anticholinergics

    c. Cholinergics

    d. Beta-adrenergic blockers

36. Which drug does *not* exert an anti-inflammatory effect?

    a. Aspirin

    b. Ibuprofen

    c. Acetaminophen

    d. COX-2 inhibitors

37. Which body system would most likely be adversely affected during high-dose aspirin therapy?

    a. GI

    b. Cardiovascular

    c. Endocrine

    d. Nervous

38. What is the primary advantage of using the selective COX-2 inhibitors over aspirin?

    a. They are less expensive.

    b. They are more efficacious.

    c. They have fewer adverse effects on the digestive system.

    d. They have greater anticoagulant ability.

39. If administrated over a long period, which class of drugs has the potential to suppress the normal functions of the adrenal gland?

    a. NSAIDs

    b. H_2-receptor antagonists

    c. Immunosuppressants

    d. Glucocorticoids

40. Which drug class is most effective at relieving severe inflammation?

    a. NSAIDs

    b. Systemic glucocorticoids

    c. H_2-receptor antagonists

    d. COX-2 inhibitors

41. In addition to its use in reducing allergy symptoms, what is diphenhydramine (Benadryl) occasionally used to treat?

    a. Mild to moderate pain

    b. Parkinson's disease

    c. Depression

    d. ADD

MAKING CONNECTIONS

42. Which route would potentially result in the most severe adverse effects?

    a. PO

    b. IV

    c. IM

    d. SC

43. For which condition is phenytoin (Dilantin) most frequently used?

    a. Bipolar disorder

    b. Migraines

    c. Schizophrenia

    d. Seizures

44. Which organ is responsible for the first-pass effect?

    a. Liver

    b. Brain

    c. Kidneys

    d. Small intestine

45. Which of the following is an opioid?

    a. Hydralazine

    b. Hydrocortisone

    c. Hydrocodone

    d. Hydrochlorothiazide

CALCULATIONS

46. A mother is to give her son Tylenol 30 gtts PO every 4 hours for elevated temperature. How many milliliters would she give her son in one dose? What would be the total gtts and milliliters given in 24-hours?

47. A physician has prescribed naproxen for stiff and painful joints. The order reads "Naprosyn 500 mg PO qid." The pharmacy sends 250 mg tablets. How many tablet(s) would the patient receive in one dose? How many milligrams will he receive in a 24-hour period, and would the amount be within the recommended dosage for a 24-hour period?

CASE STUDY APPLICATIONS

48. Mr. E is an 18-year-old patient who presents to the ED on a Sunday complaining of a severe toothache. During examination, the nurse notes an abscess surrounding a molar that is red, swollen, and inflamed. The patient also presents with a temperature of 39°C. Based on the presenting symptoms, the ARNP suspects a systemic bacterial infection, and prescribes the following medications:

    Ampicillin

    Empirin 2

    Ketoprofen (Orudis)

The inhouse pharmacy fills the prescriptions, but assigns the patient education related to drug therapy to you as the nurse in charge of the outpatient. What are your goals for this patient in regard to education?

a. Explain the therapeutic rationale for Empirin 2 and ketoprofen.

b. Explain why the ARNP did not prescribe a corticosteroid to reduce the inflammation.

c. Explain the most common adverse reactions to Empirin 2 and ketoprofen.

49. B.B. is a 64-year-old female that has been complaining of stiff and painful joints in both hands. The doctor has prescribed Celebrex. The patient education for this condition should include potential adverse reactions to the class of medications and when to notify the physician in relationship to these adverse reactions. The patient should also receive information on nonpharmacologic methods to reduce symptoms of the condition.

a. Determine the drug classification.

b. Why are the medications in this drug class the drugs of choice for treatment of inflammation?

c. What conditions should the RN assess the patient for prior to the patient receiving any drug from this classification?

50. Ms. C has brought her 6-month-old son into the ER with a temperature of 103.7°F. The physician orders Tylenol infant drops to reduce the temperature. Ms. C is a 17-year-old, first-time mother without a support system at home. She looks to the RN for information on the proper method to administer the medication to her son.

a. Why did the physician order Tylenol and not aspirin?

b. Why did the physician order infant drops?

c. What disorder can be acquired in young children with aspirin therapy?

CHAPTER 32

DRUGS FOR BACTERIAL INFECTIONS

OBJECTIVES

To view the objectives, please refer to the textbook, student CD-ROM, and the Companion Website at *www.prenhall.com/adams*.

FILL IN THE BLANK

From the textbook, find the correct word(s) to complete the statement(s).

1. The ability of an organism to cause infection is referred to as

   _____.

2. Technically, _____ refers to natural substances produced by microorganisms that can kill other microorganisms. Drugs responsible for killing infectious microorganisms are called _____.

3. Genetic errors referred to as _____ commonly occur in bacterial cells and result in drug resistance.

4. _____ infections are acquired in a hospital setting.

5. When anti-infectives are used against a wide variety of microorganisms, they are classified as

   _____.

6. _____ occurs secondarily to anti-infective therapy.

7. An enzyme secreted by bacteria that limits the therapeutic usefulness of penicillins is _____.

8. _____ are a widely prescribed class of antibiotics, similar in structure and function to the penicillins.

9. _____ antibiotics are safer alternatives to penicillin because they can generally be administered over a shorter time.

10. Narrow-spectrum antibiotics classified as _____ are useful for the treatment of serious gram-negative infections, but they also have the potential for producing ear and kidney toxicity.

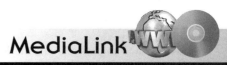

MediaLink

www.prenhall.com/adams

CD-ROM
Animation:
   Mechanism in Action: Penicillin
Audio Glossary
NCLEX Review
Companion Website
NCLEX Review
Dosage Calculations
Case Study
Care Plans
Expanded Key Concepts

MATCHING

For questions 11 through 21, match the type of medication in column I with its pharmacologic category in column II.

Column I	Column II
11. _____ Amoxicillin (Amoxil)	a. Penicillin
12. _____ Ciprofloxacin (Cipro)	b. Cephalosporin
13. _____ Cefepime (Maxipime)	c. Tetracycline
14. _____ Gentamicin sulfate (Garamycin)	d. Macrolide
15. _____ Neomycin sulfate (Mycifradin)	e. Aminoglycoside
16. _____ Erythromycin (E-mycin)	f. Fluoroquinolone or miscellaneous
17. _____ Doxycycline hyclate (Doryx)	g. Antitubercular agent
18. _____ Cephalexin (Keflex)	
19. _____ Ampicillin (Polycillin)	
20. _____ Rifampin (Rifadin, Rimactane)	
21. _____ Vancomycin (Vancocin)	

For questions 22 through 29, match the organism in column I with its disease(s) in column II.

Column I	Column II
22. _____ *Vibrio*	a. Venereal disease, endometriosis
23. _____ *Streptococci*	b. Cholera
24. _____ *Pneumococci*	c. Traveler's diarrhea, UTI, bacteremia, endometriosis
25. _____ *Rickettsia*	d. Pharyngitis, pneumonia, skin infections, septicemia, endocarditis
26. _____ *Klebsiella*	
27. _____ *Borrelia*	e. Lyme disease
28. _____ *Escherichia*	f. Rocky Mountain spotted fever
29. _____ *Chlamydia*	g. Pneumonia, otitis media, meningitis, bacteremia, endocarditis
	h. Pneumonia, UTI

MULTIPLE CHOICE

30. What is the value of using an antibiotic that is classified as a broad-spectrum antibiotic?

   a. It produces a large number of side effects.

   b. It is effective against a small number of organisms.

   c. It is effective against a large number of organisms.

   d. It has a high potency.

31. What is the action of bacteriocidal drugs?

    a. They have a high potency.

    b. They have high efficacy.

    c. They kill the infectious agent.

    d. They slow the growth of the infectious agent.

32. What is the advantage of using amoxicillin (Amoxil) over penicillin G?

    a. Less expensive

    b. Greater absorption

    c. Fewer side effects

    d. Penicillinase resistance

33. Which class of antibiotics is usually reserved for urinary tract infections and have serious adverse effects on hearing and kidney function?

    a. Erythromycin

    b. Aminoglycoside

    c. Tetracycline

    d. Sulfonamide

34. Which antibiotic is known as the "last chance" drug, for treatment of resistant infections?

    a. Clarithromycin (Biaxin)

    b. Dicloxacillin (Dynapen)

    c. Vancomycin (Vancocin)

    d. Trimethoprim-sulfamethoxazole (Septra)

35. Which antibiotic would most likely be used for the dental client allergic to penicillin?

    a. Clindamycin (Cleocin)

    b. Amoxicillin (Amoxil)

    c. Sulfisoxazole (Gantrisin)

    d. Erythromycin (E-mycin)

36. Which drug is effective against a large number of different species of bacteria?

    a. Bacteriocidal

    b. Bacteriostatic

    c. Wide spectrum

    d. Narrow spectrum

37. Photosensitivity and teeth discoloration are potential adverse effects with which of the following?

    a. Aminoglycosides

    b. Metronidazole (Flagyl)

    c. Cephalosporins

    d. Tetracyclines

38. Which is the drug of choice for the treatment of *M. tuberculosis*?

    a. Erythromycin (E-mycin, Erythrocin)

    b. Gentamicin (Garamycin)

    c. Vancomycin (Vancocin)

    d. Isoniazid (INH)

39. Which is an antibiotic responsible for causing red-man syndrome as a side effect?

    a. Cefotaxime (Claforan)

    b. Tetracycline HCl (Achromycin, others)

    c. Erythromycin (E-mycin, Erythrocin)

    d. Vancomycin (Vancocin)

40. How does drug therapy of tuberculosis differ from that of most other infections?

    a. Clients with tuberculosis have no symptoms.

    b. Mycobacteria have a cell wall that is resistant to penetration by anti-infective drugs.

    c. Clients usually require therapy for a shorter time.

    d. Antituberculosis drugs are used extensively for treating the disease, not preventing it.

41. What is the purpose of culture and sensitivity testing?

    a. To prevent an infection, a practice called chemoprophylaxis

    b. To determine which antibiotic is most effective against the infecting microorganism

    c. To identify bacteria that have acquired resistance

    d. To promote the development of drug-resistant bacterial strains by killing the bacteria sensitive to a drug

42. Which of the following types of antibiotics are more likely to cause superinfections?

    a. Narrow-spectrum antibiotics

    b. Broad-spectrum antibiotics

    c. Original penicillin

    d. Bacteriostatic drugs

43. Which antibiotic class is most widely used because of its higher margin of safety and effectiveness?

    a. Penicillins

    b. Tetracyclines

    c. Macrolides

    d. Aminoglycosides

44. Which of the following factors contribute to acquired resistance?

    a. Errors during replication of bacterial DNA

    b. Overuse of antibiotics

    c. Not taking antibiotic therapy for the prescribed length of time

    d. Both a and b

MAKING CONNECTIONS

45. Which local anesthetic drug might interfere with the antibacterial activity of some sulfonamide drugs?

    a. Benzocaine (Americaine)

    b. Tetracaine (Pontocaine)

    c. Bupivacaine (Marcaine)

    d. Lidocaine (Xylocaine)

46. Which action might influence antibiotic absorption within the stomach?

    a. Taking an antacid along with the antibiotic

    b. Drinking a glass of water with the antibiotic

    c. Taking an antibiotic suspension without shaking up the medicine vial

    d. Taking the antibiotic just before going to bed

47. If convulsive seizures were to develop with antibiotic therapy, which symptoms would most likely *not* be observed?

    a. Jerking muscular movements

    b. Difficulty breathing and biting the tongue

    c. Blank stare with psychotic symptoms

    d. Loss of bladder control

48. Following oral administration, chlorpromazine (Thorazine) is rapidly inactivated by the liver. What is this inactivation called?

    a. Enterohepatic recirculation

    b. First-pass effect

    c. Gastric-hepatic barrier

    d. Enzyme induction

49. Which term is *not* associated with the drug levodopa (Dopar)?

    a. Anticholinergic

    b. Anti-Parkinson's agent

    c. Dopamine

    d. Sympathomimetic

CALCULATIONS

50. A patient is to receive amoxicillin 500 mg PO every 6 hours for 7 days. The pharmacy sends to the floor amoxicillin 1 g in scored tablets. How many tablet(s) will the patient receive each dose? How many tablet(s) will the patient receive in a 12-hour period?

51. A patient is receiving Cipro for a urinary tract infection (UTI). The order reads: Cipro 500 mg PO qid for 5 days. The pharmacy sends Cipro 250 mg. How many tablet(s) will the patient receive in a 24-hour period?

CASE STUDY APPLICATIONS

52. For several years Ms. P has taken antibiotics on a frequent basis for kidney infections. She has been informed that she is likely to develop a drug-resistant infection. Determine possible reasons why she has reoccurring kidney infections and suggest interventions to reduce the reoccurrence of the problem.

    a. What are the potential results of the widespread use of antibiotics?

    b. What is the relationship between the long-term use of antibiotics and resistant strains of bacteria?

    c. What is the potential problem that Ms. P may develop?

    d. What will happen to the therapeutic effect of the antibiotic?

53. Mr. N has been diagnosed with bacterial pneumonia and has been treated with a broad-spectrum antibiotic until the bacteria can be isolated and the appropriate drug administered. The patient asks the RN the rationale for starting him on one antibiotic when the drug therapy may be changed after lab results have isolated the bacteria.

    a. Why are broad-spectrum antibiotics sometimes prescribed?

    b. What tests must be done to identify the microbe?

    c. What changes in treatment will be recommended after the microbe is identified?

54. Mr. K is an 88-year-old patient with impaired renal function who has been diagnosed with a urinary tract infection (UTI). He has been receiving a sulfonamide. His primary healthcare provider has determined that this is not an appropriate course of treatment for Mr. K. Examine the factors that support this decision and the potential adverse effects that might be expected if the treatment continues.

    a. What are the potential adverse effects of sulfonamides?

    b. What is the nurse's role in sulfonamide therapy?

    c. How does sulfonamide therapy affect the patient's intake of fluids?

CHAPTER 33

DRUGS FOR FUNGAL, PROTOZOAN, AND HELMINTH INFECTIONS

OBJECTIVES

To view the objectives, please refer to the textbook, student CD-ROM, and the Companion Website at *www.prenhall.com/adams*.

FILL IN THE BLANK

From the text book, find the correct word(s) to complete the statement(s).

1. _____ are single-celled or multicellular organisms that are more complex than bacteria.

2. Patients with intact immune defenses are afflicted with community-acquired infections such as

   _____, _____, _____, and _____.

3. Fungal infections acquired in a nosocomial setting will more likely be _____, _____,

   _____, and _____.

4. Fungal diseases are referred to as _____.

5. Superficial fungal infections are sometimes referred to as _____.

6. Systemic mycoses typically affect the _____, _____, and _____.

7. Some of the newer antifungal agents may be used for either _____ or _____ infections.

8. The largest class of antifungals, _____, inhibits _____ synthesis, causing the fungal plasma membrane to become porous or leaky.

9. _____ was the drug of choice for many years in the treatment of systemic fungal infections.

10. The major advantage of the azoles is that they may be administered _____.

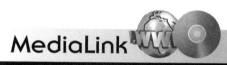

MediaLink
www.prenhall.com/adams
CD-ROM
Audio Glossary
NCLEX Review
Companion Website
NCLEX Review
Dosage Calculations
Care Plans
Expanded Key Concepts

MATCHING

For questions 11 through 16, match the name of the fungus in column I with whether it usually causes a systemic or topical infection in column II.

Column I	Column II
11. _____ *Aspergillus fumigatus*	a. Systemic infection
12. _____ *Epidermophyton floccosum*	b. Topical infection
13. _____ *Coccidioides immitis*	
14. _____ *Histoplasma capsulatum*	
15. _____ *Sporothrix schenckii*	
16. _____ *Mucorales*	

For questions 17 through 22, match the antifungal drug in column I with its indication in column II.

Column I	Column II
17. _____ Butoconazole (Femstat)	a. Skin mycoses
18. _____ Econazole nitrate (Spectazole)	b. Ringworm, skin, and nail infections
19. _____ Flucytosine (Ancobon)	c. Vaginal mycoses
20. _____ Griseofulvin (Fulvicin)	d. Severe systemic infections
21. _____ Nystatin (Mycostatin, others)	e. Candidiasis
22. _____ Undecylenic acid (Cruex, Desenex)	f. Athletes foot, diaper rash

MULTIPLE CHOICE

23. Systemic mycoses are frequently quite severe and affect more than one body system. These mycoses often require which treatment(s)?

    a. Topical agents only

    b. Oral medications only

    c. Parenteral medications only

    d. Oral and parenteral medications

24. Some systemic antifungal drugs are included in the treatment regimen of disorders not related to a fungal infection. Which disorder applies to this situation?

    a. Extensive burns

    b. Cancer

    c. Organ transplants

    d. Influenza

25. Which drug is not in widespread use for systemic fungal infections?

    a. Fluconazole (Diflucan)

    b. Itraconazole (Sporonox)

    c. Ketoconazole (Nizoral)

    d. Amphotericin B (Fungizone)

26. Candidiasis affects the skin, vagina, and mouth. Which drug is used to treat this condition and is available in a wide variety of formulations including cream, ointment, powder, tablets, and lozenges.

    a. Butenafine (Mentax)

    b. Ciclopirox olamine (Loprox)

    c. Nystatin (Mycostatin)

    d. Haloprogin (Halotex)

27. Which is the most common side effect of systemic amphotericin B therapy?

    a. Phlebitis

    b. Neurotoxicity

    c. Gastric reflux

    d. Dryness of the mouth

28. Superficial antifungal drugs are ineffective in which disorder?

    a. Nail infection

    b. Infections of the mucous membranes

    c. Suppressed immune system

    d. Infection of the scalp and hair

29. Which medication would more likely be used in the treatment of travelers' diarrhea, a condition caused by protozoans that thrive in Africa, South America, and Asia?

    a. Doxycycline hyclate (Vibramycin)

    b. Mebendazole (Vermox)

    c. Chloroquine (Aralen)

    d. Metronidazole (Flagyl)

30. Which medication was for over 60 years considered the drug of choice for the treatment of malaria? (This drug has been replaced by other antimalarials due to the frequency of resistance.)

    a. Praziquantel (Biltricide)

    b. Chloroquine (Aralen)

    c. Melarsoprol (Arsobal)

    d. Trimetrexate (Neutrexin)

31. Which organ(s) does amebiasis invade and frequently cause severe ulcers and/or abscesses?

    a. Large intestine and liver

    b. Small intestine

   c. Heart

   d. Kidney and heart

32. What is the drug of choice for the treatment of most forms of amebiasis?

   a. Mebendazole (Vermox)

   b. Amphotericin (Fungizone)

   c. Metronidazole (Flagyl)

   d. Chloroquine (Aralen)

33. What is the drug of choice for the treatment of a wide range of helminth infections?

   a. Mebendazole (Vermox)

   b. Amphotericin (Fungizone)

   c. Metronidazole (Flagyl)

   d. Chloroquine (Aralen)

34. Patient education for the treatment of helminths should include which of the following?

   a. Instruct the patient to stop the drug therapy as soon as he or she feels better.

   b. Instruct the patient that all family members need to be treated at the same time to prevent reinfestation.

   c. Instruct the patient to wear tight underwear.

   d. Instruct the patient not to wash bedding until drug regime is completed.

35. What sociologic factor would the nurse need to evaluate in relationship to parasitic infections?

   a. Upper-middle-class lifestyle

   b. Good personal hygiene

   c. Poverty level income

   d. Single-parent family

MAKING CONNECTIONS

36. During the mutation of infectious agents, what part of their physical makeup is altered?

   a. DNA

   b. Protein

   c. Beta-lactam ring

   d. Enzymes

37. Which drug or class of drugs induces hepatic microsomal enzymes, decreasing the effectiveness of some antiparasitic medications?

   a. Opioids

   b. Phenobarbital

   c. Aspirin

   d. Phenothiazines

38. A drug that increases the renal reabsorption of an antiviral medication also would do which of the following?

    a. Increase the half-life of the medication

    b. Decrease the half-life of the medication

    c. Have no effect on the half-life of the medication

    d. Also increase excretion

39. A patient who is allergic to penicillin G has the potential to be allergic to which of the following?

    a. Ampicillin (Polycillin)

    b. Tetracycline

    c. Ciprofloxacin (Cipro)

    d. Vancomycin (Vancocin)

40. To what drug classification does ibuprofen belong?

    a. Salicylate

    b. Opioid

    c. Selective COX-2 inhibitor

    d. NSAID

CALCULATIONS

41. The physician has ordered amphotericin B, 0.25 mg/kg qd for the patient, who weighs 150 lb. What is the patient's weight in kg? How many mg of medication will the patient receive a day?

42. Diflucan has been ordered to treat a patient's yeast infection. The order reads 200 mg PO on day 1 to be followed by 100 mg PO qd for a total drug regime of 2 weeks. What is the total number of mg the patient will receive daily after day 1?

CASE STUDY APPLICATIONS

43. Mrs. B is 38 weeks' pregnant and displays the symptoms of vaginal candidiasis. The apparent infection is not serious, but it is a concern to the nurse. Patient education regarding treatment is a priority for this patient related to the pregnancy.

    a. What approach should Mrs. B take to have this infection treated?

    b. What precautions should be considered during the treatment?

44. Mr. C has just returned from an extended trip to South America and has been diagnosed with malaria. The primary nursing consideration for this patient is education monitoring for potential adverse reactions to the drug therapy.

    a. What is the recommended drug regimen for malaria?

    b. What are the potential adverse reactions to the recommended drug regimen?

45. Mrs. G has also returned from an extended vacation in Latin America and displays the symptoms of amebiasis. The RN must understand the progression of this disease to carefully monitor this patient's condition. The RN must also be sure that the patient receives education in relationship to her drug regimen.

    a. What drug regimen will the patient receive for this condition?

    b. What are the most common adverse reactions to this drug regimen?

    c. Primarily this is a disease of what organ of the body?

CHAPTER 34

DRUGS FOR VIRAL INFECTIONS

OBJECTIVES

To view the objectives, please refer to the textbook, student CD-ROM, and the Companion Website at *www.prenhall.com/adams*.

FILL IN THE BLANK

From the textbook, find the correct word(s) to complete the statement(s).

1. The basic structure of a virus includes the outer protein coat or the _____, and the inner genetic materials in the form of _____ or _____.

2. Viruses are considered _____, therefore they require a host to replicate.

3. During the _____ stage, the patient is asymptomatic and may not be aware of the HIV infection.

4. The classification of medications used to block components of the replication cycle of human immunodeficiency virus (HIV) is _____.

5. The standard aggressive treatment for HIV-AIDS using as many as four drugs concurrently is called _____.

6. Oseltamivir (Tamiflu) and zanamivir (Relenza) are examples of a newer classification of drugs called the _____ and are used to treat active influenza infection.

7. Agenerase is classified as a (an) _____.

8. Hepatitis B (HBV) is caused by a _____ virus and is transmitted primarily through exposure to _____ and _____.

9. _____ is the drug most often used for the treatment of herpes virus.

10. Rebetron is currently used for the treatment of chronic _____ infection.

MATCHING

For questions 11 through 15, match the description in column I with the term in column II.

Column I	Column II
11. _____ Nucleoside reverse transcriptase inhibitors	a. HAART
12. _____ Nonnucleoside reverse transcriptase inhibitors	b. Capsid
	c. NRTI
13. _____ Protein coat	d. NNRTI
14. _____ Mature infective particle	e. Virion
15. _____ Highly active antiretroviral therapy	

MULTIPLE CHOICE

16. Which drug used to treat HIV/AIDS is a nonnucleoside reverse transcriptase inhibitor?

    a. Zidovudine (Retrovir, AZT)

    b. Nevirapine (Viramune)

    c. Lamivudine (Epivir, 3TC)

    d. Indinavir sulfate (Crixivan)

17. Acyclovir (Zovirax) is not an effective treatment for which virus?

    a. Herpes simplex viruses (HSV) types 1 and 2

    b. Cytomegalovirus (CMV)

    c. Varicella-zoster virus

    d. Epstein-Barr virus

18. Which is the best approach to influenza treatment?

    a. Prevention through annual vaccinations

    b. Amantadine (Symmetrel)

    c. Oseltamivir (Tamiflu)

    d. Zanamivir (Relenza)

19. The purpose and expected outcome of HIV pharmacotherapy includes which of the following?

    a. Patients with HIV are able to live symptom-free much longer.

    b. The FDA has approved over 16 new antiviral drugs for the cure of HIV.

    c. Drugs have been developed that treat only slowly mutating and less-resistant HIV strains.

    d. Drugs have become available that treat the HIV-infected mother without much success to the newborn.

20. What is the purpose of highly active antiretroviral therapy (HAART)?

    a. To eliminate the virus from the blood

    b. To isolate HIV to the lymph nodes

    c. To reduce the plasma level of HIV to its lowest possible value

    d. All of the above

21. Which class of antivirials has most recently been discovered?

    a. Nonnucleoside reverse transcriptase inhibitors (NNRTIs)

    b. Nucleoside reverse transcriptase inhibitors (NRTIs)

    c. Fusion inhibitors

    d. DNA synthesis inhibitor

22. What is a major adverse effect of zidovudine (Retrovir, AZT)?

    a. Reduced numbers of red and white blood cells

    b. Painful inflammation of blood vessels at the site of infusion

    c. Nephrotoxicity

    d. Both b and c

23. The nurse should instruct the patient receiving NRTIs to report which adverse effects?

    a. Rash, abdominal pain, nausea, vomiting, numbness, or burning of the feet or hands

    b. Fever, chills, blistering of the skin, reddening of the skin, muscle or joint pain

    c. Headache, insomnia, fever, constipation, cough, fainting, or visual changes

    d. None of the above

24. The nurse should instruct the patient receiving NNRTIs to report which adverse effects?

    a. Rash, abdominal pain, nausea, vomiting, numbness, or burning of the feet or hands

    b. Fever, chills, blistering of the skin, reddening of the skin, muscle or joint pain

    c. Headache, insomnia, fever, constipation, cough, fainting, or visual changes

    d. None of the above

25. The nurse should instruct the patient receiving protease inhibitors to report which adverse effects?

    a. Rash, abdominal pain, nausea, vomiting, numbness, or burning of the feet or hands

    b. Fever, chills, blistering of the skin, reddening of the skin, muscle or joint pain

    c. Headache, insomnia, fever, constipation, cough, fainting, or visual changes

    d. None of the above

26. When a virus mutates, which molecules are altered?

    a. RNA or DNA

    b. Beta-lactam ring

    c. Enzymes

    d. Protein

MAKING CONNECTIONS

27. Which drugs or class of drugs induces hepatic microsomal enzymes, resulting in drug-drug interactions?

    a. Aspirin

    b. Phenobarbital

    c. Phenothiazines

    d. Opioids

28. A drug that increases the renal reabsorption of antiviral medication would have what affect?

    a. Increase the half-life of the antiviral

    b. Decrease the half-life of the antiviral

    c. Have no effect on the half-life of the antiviral

    d. Also increase excretion

29. A patient who is allergic to penicillin G will most likely also be allergic to which of the following?

    a. Tetracycline

    b. Vancomycin

    c. Ampicillin

    d. Ciprofloxacin

30. Naproxen (Naprosyn) is classified as which of the following?

    a. Salicylate

    b. Selective COX-2 inhibitor

    c. Opioid

    d. NSAID

CALCULATIONS

31. Mrs. V is to receive amantadine (Symmetrel) 100 mg PO bid × 5 days for an episode of influenza. The pharmacy has only 50 mg tablets on hand. How many tablets would Mrs. V receive per dose? How many tablets would she receive per day?

32. Mr. X is to receive 9 mcg Infergen SC three times/week × 24 weeks for hepatitis B. The pharmacy has only Infergen 20 mcg/ml in stock. How many milliliters would he receive and what type syringe would be used to measure the medication?

CASE STUDY APPLICATIONS

33. Mr. R is HIV positive and was told that combination drug therapy would be more effective for this disorder than a single drug. The RN should include in the patient education the rationale behind this type of drug therapy, the class of the drugs, and their individual actions. The RN must remember that patient education must be explained in terms that the patient can understand.

    a. Why is combination drug therapy more effective against HIV?

b. What are the drugs classes used in the combination therapy?

c. What is the action of each drug?

34. Mrs. B is pregnant with her first child and is in her third trimester. Her delivery date is late fall. Her physician has recommended that she take the influenza vaccination. Assess the rationale for this recommendation based on the information known at this time.

a. What is the rationale for her physician recommending the influenza vaccination?

b. How long is the vaccination effective?

c. Which antiviral drug has been used for many years to prevent and treat influenza?

35. Mr. C, a nurse, has been diagnosed with hepatitis B. His physician has informed him, that this disease causes inflammation and necrosis of the liver. The RN in charge of patient education for Mr. C has determined that he should be aware of symptoms displayed with his condition and also how it can be transmitted to others.

a. How is this disease transmitted?

b. What are the symptoms displayed with acute hepatitis B?

c. What are the symptoms displayed with chronic hepatitis B?

d. What is the current recommendation for the hepatitis B vaccination?

36. Ms. M has been diagnosed with genital herpes. She also is 3 months' pregnant. The RN in charge of this patient must be aware of the potential adverse reactions of most medications in relationship to pregnancy.

a. Should the physician prescribe an antiviral medication for her at this time?

b. What antiviral would mostly likely be recommended for genital herpes if the answer to question a is yes?

c. What two major adverse effects are known to be associated with this drug?

CHAPTER 35

DRUGS FOR NEOPLASIA

OBJECTIVES

To view the objectives please refer to the textbook, student CD-ROM, and the Companion Website at *www.prenhall.com/adams*.

FILL IN THE BLANK

From the textbook, find the correct word(s) to complete the statement(s).

1. Factors called _____ have been found to cause cancer or are associated with a higher risk for acquiring the disease.

2. Abnormal genes that promote cancer formation in patients are called _____.

3. One type of drug therapy for cancer is _____.

4. Treatment strategies found to increase the effectiveness of anticancer drugs include _____, _____, _____, and _____.

5. Bone marrow suppression is a major adverse effect of a class of drugs called _____.

6. By blocking the synthesis of _____, methotrexate (Mexate) inhibits replication in rapidly dividing cancer cells.

7. Most antitumor antibiotics are administered _____ or through direct installation into a body cavity using a catheter.

8. Vinca alkaloids, taxoids, and topoisomerase inhibitors are classified as _____.

9. A natural class of antineoplastic medications referred to as _____ and _____ antagonists have fewer cytoxic effects than seen with other antitumor medication.

10. _____ modifiers assist in limiting the severe immunosuppressive effects of other anticancer drugs by stimulating the body's immune system.

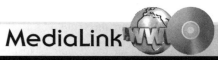

MediaLink

www.prenhall.com/adams

CD-ROM
Animation:
    Mechanism in Action: Methotrexate
    (Mexate)
Audio Glossary
NCLEX Review

Companion Website
NCLEX Review
Dosage Calculations
Case Study
Care Plans
Expanded Key Concepts

MATCHING

For questions 11 through 17, match the type of tumor in column I with its location in the body in column II.

Column I	**Column II**
11. _____ Adenoma	a. Lymphatic tissue
12. _____ Lipoma	b. Central nervous system
13. _____ Leukemia	c. Bone, muscle, and cartilage
14. _____ Lymphoma	d. Glandular tissue
15. _____ Glioma	e. Adipose tissue
16. _____ Sarcoma	f. Skin
17. _____ Melanoma	g. Blood-forming cells in bone marrow

For questions 18 through 27, match the medication in column I with its pharmacologic category in column II.

Column I	**Column II**
18. _____ Cyclophosphamide (Cytoxan, Neosar)	a. Alkylating agents
19. _____ Fluorouracil (5-FU, Adrucil, others)	b. Antimetabolites
20. _____ Vincristine sulfate (Oncovin)	c. Antitumor antibiotics
21. _____ Methotrexate (Amethopterin, others)	d. Hormones and hormone antagonists
22. _____ Bleomycin sulfate (Blenoxane)	e. Plant extracts
23. _____ Medroxyprogesterone (Provera, Depo-Provera)	f. Biologic response modifiers and miscellaneous
24. _____ Etoposide (VePesid)	
25. _____ Tamoxifen citrate (Nolvadex)	
26. _____ Levamisole (Ergamisol)	
27. _____ Streptozocin (Zanosar)	

MULTIPLE CHOICE

28. What is the mechanism of action of antimetabolites in the treatment of neoplasia?

   a. Changing the structure of DNA in cancer cells

   b. Disrupting critical cell pathways in cancer cells

   c. Preventing cell division

   d. Activating the body's immune system

29. Abnormal genes involved in the promotion of cancer formation are referred to as which of the following?

   a. Oncogenes

   b. Tumor suppressing genes

   c. Carcinogens

   d. Palliation genes

30. The nurse should instruct the patient to implement which changes in lifestyle to reduce the probability of acquiring cancer?

    a. Examining the skin for abnormal lesions or changes to moles

    b. Exercising regularly and keeping body weight within normal guidelines

    c. Examining the body monthly for abnormal lumps

    d. All of the above

31. Which food(s) are *not* considered to exert protective effects against cancer?

    a. Coldwater fish

    b. Fresh fruits and vegetables

    c. Olive oil

    d. Grains and cereals

32. Which approach has a goal of eliminating 100% of cancer cells and reducing toxicity?

    a. Using multiple drugs in lower doses from different antineoplastic classes

    b. Increasing the concentration of different antineoplastic drugs

    c. Increasing the dose of one type of antineoplastic drug

    d. Combining radiation therapy with chemotherapy treatment

33. Which problem is *not* an expected adverse effect of chemotherapy?

    a. Alopecia

    b. Nausea

    c. Hypercholesterolemia

    d. Leukopenia

34. Which drug changes the shape of DNA and prevents it from functioning normally?

    a. Cyclophosphamide (Cytoxan)

    b. Methotrexate (Mexate)

    c. Doxorubicin (Adriamycin)

    d. Vincristine (Oncovin)

35. Which is the primary drug for AIDS-related Kaposi's sarcoma?

    a. Mechlorethamine (Mustargen)

    b. Floxuridine (FUDR)

    c. Doxorubicin (Adriamycin)

    d. Teniposide (Vumon)

36. Which chemotherapeutic agent is a natural product from the Pacific yew plant?

    a. Mercaptopurine (6-MP, Purinethol)

    b. Paclitaxel (Taxol)

    c. Vinblastine sulfate (Velban)

    d. Flutamide (Eulexin)

37. Which is the most serious adverse effect to vincristine (Oncovin)?

    a. Flulike symptoms

    b. Hepatotoxicity

    c. Neurotoxicity

    d. Immunosuppression

38. Which is the drug of choice for treating breast cancer?

    a. Carboplatin (Paraplatin)

    b. Pentostatin (Nipent)

    c. Epirubicin (Ellence)

    d. Tamoxifen citrate (Nolvadex)

39. Which anticancer drug has a similar chemical structure to the insecticide DDT?

    a. Interferon alfa-2 (Roferon-A, Intron A)

    b. Mitotane (Lysodren)

    c. Paclitaxel (Taxol)

    d. Irinotecan (Camptosar)

40. Which drug might be given for palliation of cancer in the advanced stages?

    a. Epirubicin (Ellence)

    b. Dacarbazine (DTIC-Dome)

    c. Ethinyl estradiol (Estinyl)

    d. Chlorambucil (Leukeran)

41. Which drug would *not* be used in the treatment of prostate cancer?

    a. Vinorelbine tartrate (Navelbine)

    b. Megestrol acetate (Megace)

    c. Bicalutamide (Casodex)

    d. Leuprolide acetate (Lupron)

42. Which drug most likely would be used for palliative treatment of malignant melanoma?

    a. Teniposide (Vumon)

    b. Idarubicin (Idamycin)

    c. Dactinomycin (Actinomycin-D, Cosmegen)

    d. Hydroxyurea (Hydrea)

43. Which drug class would most likely displace an antineoplastic drug from protein-binding sites in the plasma, increasing its effect?

    a. NSAIDs

    b. Sedative-hypnotics

    c. Antidepressants

    d. Calcium channel blockers

MAKING CONNECTIONS

44. Heart failure is sometimes observed with antineoplastic drugs. Which symptoms would be observed in this patient?

    a. Hypokalemia

    b. Peripheral edema

    c. Dehydration

    d. Dysrhythmias

45. What are glycoprotein IIb/IIIa inhibitors used to treat?

    a. Blood coagulation disorders

    b. Depression

    c. Tuberculosis

    d. HIV/AIDS

46. Valproic acid (Depakote) is used in the pharmacotherapy of migraines, bipolar disorder, and which of the following?

    a. Schizophrenia

    b. Angina

    c. Dysrhythmias

    d. Seizures

47. Indomethacin (Indocin) is a medication that prevents prostaglandin synthesis. It is most commonly used in the treatment of which of the following?

    a. Fungal infections

    b. Pain and inflammation

    c. Hypotension

    d. Alzheimer's disease

CALCULATIONS

48. A patient is to receive tamoxifen 20 mg qd for the treatment of metastatic breast cancer. The medication is only available in 10 mg form. How many tablets would the patient receive per dose?

49. A patient has begun to experience periods of nausea and vomiting as an adverse reaction to the tamoxifen therapy. The order reads Compazine 25 mg IM q6h PRN for nausea and/or vomiting. The pharmacy has only Compazine 50 mg/2ml available. How many milliliters should the patient receive total per day?

CASE STUDY APPLICATIONS

50. Mr. U is a 40-year-old factory worker with a 10th grade education. With his early cancer of the prostate, he has been told that a drug killing 99% of tumor cells would be considered a very effective drug, but the, remaining cells could cause his tumor to return. Mr. U displays lack of understanding about his condition. As the RN assigned to his patient education, assess the situation and determine what information you would include in the following areas.

    a. Explain the treatment to prevent reoccurrence of the tumor in relationship to the stage of the tumor when the treatment began.

    b. Explain why classes of antineoplastics might be more effective than others in relationship to the cancer's stage.

    c. Explain the rationale for specific dosing schedules.

51. Ms. H has been receiving chemotherapy for 3 weeks and has experienced a number of side effects including nausea, vomiting, infections, and anorexia. She is an independent 67-year-old who chooses to remain at home alone during her treatment. As the home health nurse assigned to this case, examine possible interventions to put into place.

    a. What medications may be used to treat nausea and vomiting related to chemotherapy?

    b. What interventions may be used to lower the risk for infections?

    c. Describe the interventions for maintaining nutritional balance during chemotherapy.

52. Mrs. Y a 32-year-old schoolteacher who recently began taking tamoxifen for metastatic breast cancer and has experienced a "tumor flare." She is concerned with the outcome of this development in regard to her recovery. As the RN assigned to her, examine your patient education goals and interventions.

    a. Explain this condition in regard to the medication.

    b. Explain the classification of this drug.

    c. Explain the type of tumors this medication is effective against.

    d. Explain the unique feature of this medication.

    e. Should this medication be given during pregnancy?

CHAPTER 36

DRUGS FOR PEPTIC ULCER DISEASE

OBJECTIVES

To view the objectives, please refer to the textbook, student CD-ROM, and the Companion Website at *www.prenhall.com/adams*.

FILL IN THE BLANK

From the textbook, find the correct word(s) to complete the statement(s).

1. The digestive system consists of two basic anatomical divisions: the _____ canal and the _____ organs.

2. The primary functions of the GI tract are to physically _____ ingested food and to provide the necessary _____ and surface area for chemical _____ and _____ of nutrients into the bloodstream.

3. The small intestine is lined with tiny projections called _____ and _____ that provide a huge surface area for the absorption of _____.

4. Substances are propelled along the GI tract by the process of _____, rhythmic contraction of layers of _____ muscle.

5. The _____ prevents the stomach contents from moving backwards into the esophagus, a condition known as _____.

6. The _____ cells secrete pepsinogen and the _____ cells secrete hydrochloric acid and _____, which are essential for the absorption of vitamin B_{12}.

MediaLink

www.prenhall.com/adams

CD-ROM
Animations:
  Mechanism in Action: Ranitidine (Zantac)
Audio Glossary
NCLEX Review
Companion Website
NCLEX Review
Dosage Calculations
Case Study
Care Plans
Expanded Key Concepts

7. Gastric juice is the most _____ in the body and has a pH of _____.

8. An ulcer is a(an) _____ of the _____ layer of the GI tract; _____ is the most common site.

9. External risk factors associated with _____(PUD) include drugs, particularly _____,

   _____, and _____.

10. The primary cause of PUD is infection by the gram-negative bacterium _____.

MATCHING

For questions 11 through 17, match the correct term in column I with the definition in column II.

Column I	Column II
11. _____ GERD	a. Ulcerations in the lower small intestine
12. _____ PUD	b. Hypersecretion of gastric acid
13. _____ Crohn's disease	c. Lesion located in the stomach or small intestine
14. _____ Ulcerative colitis	
15. _____ NSAIDs	d. Increase acid secretion in the stomach
16. _____ H$_2$-receptors	e. Backward movement of stomach contents
17. _____ Zollinger-Ellison syndrome	f. Nonsteroidal anti-inflammatory drugs
	g. Erosions located in the large intestine

MULTIPLE CHOICE

18. In caring for a client with peptic ulcer disease, the healthcare provider must understand that digestive enzymes are secreted by all of the following except which one?

    a. Salivary glands

    b. Stomach

    c. Pancreas

    d. Microvilli

19. You are developing education materials for your client. Which of the following is *not* a risk factor associated with peptic ulcer disease (PUD)?

    a. Family history

    b. Blood type AB

    c. Psychological stress

    d. *H. pylori*

20. During your assessment, which characteristic symptom is most indicative of a duodenal ulcer?

    a. Gnawing or burning in the upper abdomen

    b. Nighttime pain, nausea, and vomiting

    c. Bright red blood in the stool

    d. Bright red blood in the vomitus

21. Your client has a prior history of gastric ulcers. Which of the following would be increased in the presence of a recurrence?

    a. Hunger, even after meals

    b. Frequency of remissions

    c. Frequency in 30 to 50-year age group

    d. Pain, briefly relieved by food

22. Inflammatory bowel disease (IBD) includes which of the following?

    a. Both gastric and duodenal ulcers

    b. Zollinger-Ellison syndrome

    c. Crohn's disease and ulcerative colitis

    d. PUD and GERD

23. Your client is overweight and complaining of an intense burning (heartburn) in the chest, which is indicative of which of the following conditions?

    a. PUD

    b. GERD

    c. IBD

    d. Crohn's disease

24. In developing a plan of care for your client with peptic ulcer disease, you need to include all of the following except which one?

    a. Smoking cessation

    b. Abstinence from alcohol

    c. Avoidance of caffeine

    d. Severe dietary restrictions

25. Which class of drugs reduces acid secretion in the stomach by binding irreversibly to an enzyme on the parietal cells?

    a. H_2-receptor antagonists

    b. Serotonin receptor antagonists

    c. Proton pump inhibitors

    d. Antacids

26. Which class of peptic ulcer medications consists of alkaline combinations of aluminum hydroxide and magnesium hydroxide?

    a. Phenothiazines

   b. Serotonin receptor antagonists

   c. Proton pump inhibitors

   d. Antacids

27. Which of the following best describes the mechanism of action of sucralfate (Carafate)?

   a. Kills *H. pylori*

   b. Adds a gel-like protective mucus over the ulcer

   c. Reduces secretion of acid

   d. Increases the secretion of bicarbonate

MAKING CONNECTIONS

28. Why is tetracycline (Achromycin) not used in children under 12 years?

   a. Causes penicillin-like reactions

   b. Stains forming deciduous teeth

   c. Is primarily used to treat acne

   d. Only used to treat Lyme disease

29. Clarithromycin (Biaxin) is effective against *H. pylori* because of which reason? It is

   a. Effective against gram-positive and gram-negative organisms

   b. A macrolide that can be given to people with penicillin allergies

   c. Considered to be a broad-spectrum antibiotic

   d. All of the above

30. Metronidazole (Flagyl) is all of the following except which one?

   a. Considered an antibacterial agent

   b. Effective in the treatment of STDs

   c. Classified as an aminoglycoside

   d. Used in the treatment of protozoal infections

31. Which of the following would *not* be expected from an overdose of an opioid?

   a. CNS depression

   b. Diarrhea

   c. Respiratory depression

   d. Constricted pupils

32. Mr. D is receiving a HMG-CoA reductase inhibitor. He is most likely being treated for which of the following?

   a. High lipid levels in the blood

   b. Stroke

   c. Schizophrenia

   d. Hypertension

CALCULATIONS

Your patient is to receive the following medications. Calculate the correct dosages as required.

33. Ranitidine (Zantac) 50 mg IV in 100 ml to infuse in 30 min by microdrip.

   a. How many gtt/hr is this?

   b. How many ml/hr will the nurse set the infusion pump to deliver?

34. Aluminum hydroxide (Amphojel) 2 T qid, PO.

   a. What times would the nurse give this medication?

   b. Give the correct equivalents in teaspoons, milliliters, and ounces.

CASE STUDY APPLICATIONS

35. Mr. G is an elderly patient who is admitted with a recurrence of gastric ulcers. His wife tells you that he has been taking cimetidine (Tagamet) as an OTC preparation. She tells you that he no longer complains of the gnawing pain in his stomach but has become increasingly confused within the past 3 days. During your initial assessment you note that the patient is oriented to person and time but not place.

   a. Name at least two appropriate nursing diagnoses for this patient.

   b. Prioritize your diagnoses and give your rationales.

36. You continue to care for your patient and you note that cimetidine has been discontinued by doctor's order. Your patient is now on ranitidine (Zantac).

   a. What would be your short-term goal for this patient?

   b. During the implementation of your plan for care, what laboratory values would you assess for this patient? Why?

37. While you are preparing your patient for discharge, he has been placed on omeprazole (Prilosec) and antacids. In preparing your patient education for both Mr. G and his wife related to these medications.

   a. What would be an appropriate nursing diagnosis for this couple?

   b. What basic instruction is necessary in relation to OTC medications?

   c. What does this patient need to know about the timing of his medications?

CHAPTER 37

DRUGS FOR BOWEL DISORDERS, NAUSEA, AND VOMITING

OBJECTIVES

To view the objectives, please refer to the textbook, student CD-ROM, and the Companion Website at *www.prenhall.com/adams*.

FILL IN THE BLANK

From the textbook, find the correct word(s) to complete the statement(s).

1. Psychological factors related to nausea occur during periods

   of extreme _____ or when confronted with

   unpleasant _____, _____, and

   _____.

2. The two major drug classes used to effectively treat nausea due to motion sickness are _____ and

   _____.

3. Ingestion of poisons is sometimes treated by administering _____ such as _____ to

   induce _____ within 15 minutes.

4. _____ are used for the treatment of obesity, although they produce only _____

   effects.

5. Constipation is identified by a decrease in the _____ and number of _____.

6. The etiology of constipation may be related to insufficient _____, especially insoluble

   _____.

7. Severe constipation can lead to a fecal _____ and a complete _____ of the bowel.

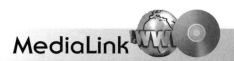

MediaLink

www.prenhall.com/adams

CD-ROM
Audio Glossary
NCLEX Review

Companion Website
NCLEX Review
Dosage Calculations
Case Study
Care Plans
Expanded Key Concepts

8. Prophylactic pharmacotherapy with _____ is appropriate to preclude straining or bearing down during _____ .

9. The role of the nurse in pharmacotherapy involves careful _____ of a patient's condition and providing _____ .

10. Laxatives are contraindicated in _____ , _____ , and _____ due to the risk for causing _____ perforation.

MATCHING

For questions 11 through 17, match the correct term in column I with the definition in column II.

Column I	**Column II**
11. _____ Laxative	a. Causes water and fat to be absorbed into stools
12. _____ Cathartic	b. Promotes defecation
13. _____ Bulk-forming agent	c. Lubricates the stool and colon
14. _____ Stool softener	d. Irritates the bowel causing peristalsis
15. _____ Stimulant	e. Absorbs water increasing size of fecal mass
16. _____ Osmotic	f. Pulls water into stool for a more watery stool
17. _____ Mineral oil	g. Implies a strong and complete bowel emptying

MULTIPLE CHOICE

18. Acting on which of the following patient complaints would the nurse discontinue laxative therapy?

   a. Nausea with dry skin

   b. Mild abdominal discomfort

   c. Diarrhea and cramping

   d. A soft formed stool

19. All of the following describe stimulant laxatives except which one?

   a. Peristalsis is increased by irritating the colon

   b. Results are both rapid and effective

   c. Never used in combination with other types

   d. Frequently used as an aid to a bowel prep

20. Patients receiving prochlorperazine (Compazine) for nausea must also be monitored for which of the following?

   a. Extrapyramidal symptoms

   b. Cholinergic side effects

   c. Early Parkinson's disease

   d. Hyperemesis gravidarum

21. Patient education should include which of the following?

    a. Goals of therapy

    b. Reason for treatment

    c. Possible side effects

    d. All of the above

22. A nursing assessment of a patient on laxative therapy should include all of the following except which one?

    a. Vital signs

    b. Abdominal assessment

    c. Level of consciousness

    d. Character of stool

23. Which of the following is a bulk-forming laxative?

    a. Psyllium mucilloid (Metamucil)

    b. Docusate sodium (Colace)

    c. Senna root

    d. Cascara sagrada

24. Aprepitant (Emend) is a new antiemetic that belongs to which of the following drug classifications?

    a. Neurokinin receptor

    b. Serotonin-receptor blockers

    c. Glucocorticoids

    d. Phenothiazines

25. Which of the following is a common complication secondary to the administration of bulk-forming laxatives?

    a. Bowel perforation

    b. Severe hypotension

    c. Stimulation of defecation

    d. Obstruction of the esophagus

26. Which of the following categories of laxatives are known for their high sodium content?

    a. Bulk forming

    b. Stimulant laxatives

    c. Osmotic laxatives

    d. Herbal laxative preparations

27. Which of the following drugs is the most widely prescribed anorexiant for short-term control of obesity?

    a. Dextroamphetamine (Dexedrine)

    b. Sibutramine (Meridia)

    c. Orlistat (Xenical)

    d. Dimenhydrinate (Dramamine)

28. Misoprostol (Cytotec) is an antiulcer agent. What nursing intervention is necessary before administering to a female of childbearing age?

    a. Checking a complete blood count (CBC)

    b. Monitoring for gastric signs and symptoms

    c. Urine for pregnancy (UCG)

    d. Testing for *H. pylori*

29. Scopolamine (Transderm-Scop) is an effective antiemetic for motion sickness. What is this drug classified as?

    a. Adrenergic agonist

    b. Cholinergic agonist

    c. Anticholinergic

    d. Ganglionic blocker

MAKING CONNECTIONS

30. An adrenergic crisis is evidenced by which of the following?

    a. Decreased heart rate

    b. Decreased respiratory rate

    c. Increased peristalsis

    d. Dilated pupils

31. Diphenhydramine (Benadryl) is an antihistamine. Which of the following is a common side effect?

    a. Headache

    b. Nasal stuffiness

    c. Drowsiness

    d. Salivation

32. Phenothiazines can cause extrapyramidal symptoms. Which of the following medications would be given to reverse this syndrome?

    a. Benzotropine (Cogentin)

    b. Atropine sulfate

    c. Midazolam (Versed)

    d. Naloxone (Narcan)

CALCULATIONS

33. Your patient is to receive prochlorperazine (Compazine) 10 mg, q4–6h, IM, PRN for relief of nausea and vomiting. The medication on hand is 25 mg per 2 ml ampule.

    a. How much of this medication will be used for each dose?

    b. What type of syringe should be used?

    c. What length and gauge needle is appropriate for this medication?

34. To control loose stools, your patient has been prescribed diphenoxylate with atropine (Lomotil). A dose of 2.5 mg, PO, qid has been ordered. How many milligrams will this patient receive in 24 hours?

CASE STUDY APPLICATIONS

35. Mr. D is admitted complaining of an inability to move his bowels for the past 5 days. You observe that his abdomen is distended; he is somewhat anxious; his vital signs are slightly elevated in comparison to those you received in report from the ED nurse. The doctor has ordered an osmotic laxative.

    a. Identify two high-priority nursing diagnoses for this patient.

    b. What are the goals related to each of these diagnoses?

    c. List at least two nursing actions that will be implemented to assist in achieving these goals.

    d. What criteria would you use to determine the effectiveness of your plan of care based on patient outcomes?

36. Mrs. W, age 82, complains of diarrhea for the past 3 days. She states she has had more than five or more liquefied stools a day during this time. She has not noted any bleeding, however. Antidiarrheal therapy has begun.

    a. As the nurse assigned to this patient, what will you include in your initial assessment?

    b. What objective data will be important for you to observe?

    c. What safety issues would need to be considered?

37. Ms. C, age 24, is admitted with severe nausea and vomiting. She tells you that she has experienced this discomfort every morning for a week. Her pregnancy test comes back positive. This condition is known as hyperemesis gravidarum. Intravenous fluids are ordered along with an antiemetic.

    a. What assessment will you make to ensure the safety of mother and fetus?

    b. What is the primary therapeutic goal for Ms. C?

    c. Prochlorperazine (Compazine) is the prototype drug of antiemetics. Would it be appropriate for this patient? If not, why?

    d. What outcome criteria will alert you to the fact that this patient's goals have been accomplished?

38. You assist with the admission of Mrs. G, 350 lb, 5'8." She is complaining of hunger, stating, "I have not eaten since yesterday." It is now noontime and dinner trays are being served. The patient tells you that she is not only "hungry" but has a "large appetite" and requests two cheeseburgers for lunch instead of the usual one that appears on her tray. You note on her admission assessment that she has been on the anorexiant orlistat (Xenical).

    a. What dietary restrictions should be part of this patient's education?

    b. What supplemental medications may be needed due to the decreased absorption of other substances?

    c. What nonpharmacologic support will supplement the care plan of this patient in relation to her "hunger," "appetite," and "weight reduction program"?

CHAPTER 38

DRUGS FOR NUTRITIONAL DISORDERS

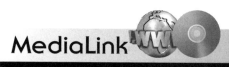

OBJECTIVES

To view the objectives, please refer to the textbook, student CD-ROM, and the Companies Website at *www.prenhall.com/adams*.

MediaLink

www.prenhall.com/adams

CD-ROM
Audio Glossary
NCLEX Review

Companion Website
NCLEX Review
Dosage Calculations
Case Study
Care Plans
Expanded Key Concepts

FILL IN THE BLANK

From the textbook, find the correct word(s) to complete the statement(s).

1. Vitamins are essential substances needed in very small _____ to maintain _____.

2. An important characteristic of vitamins is that, with the exception of vitamin _____, human cells cannot _____ them.

3. Without vitamin K, abnormal _____ is produced and _____ is affected.

4. Vitamins that dissolve in lipids are called _____ and include vitamins _____.

5. _____ vitamins cannot be absorbed in the small _____ but can be stored in large quantities in the _____ and adipose tissue.

6. Recommended _____ (_____) values represent the _____ amount of vitamin or mineral needed to prevent a _____ in a healthy adult.

7. _____ or toxic levels of vitamins have been reported for vitamins _____, _____, _____, _____, _____, _____ and _____.

8. _____ is the most common cause of _____ deficiency in the United States.

9. Vitamin D$_2$, also known as _____, is obtained from fortified milk, margarine, and other dairy products.

10. _____ is considered a primary antioxidant, preventing the formation of _____ that

damage cell _____ and other cellular structures.

MATCHING

For questions 11 through 17, match the correct term in column I with the definition in column II.

Column I	Column II
11. _____ Vitamin K	a. Problems with night vision
12. _____ Vitamins A, D, E, and K	b. Skeletal abnormalities
13. _____ Vitamin A deficiency	c. Synthesis of heme
14. _____ Vitamin D	d. Fat-soluble vitamins
15. _____ Vitamin B complex	e. Antidote for warfarin (Coumadin)
16. _____ Vitamin B$_6$	f. Folic acid
17. _____ Vitamin B$_9$	g. Twelve different vitamins

MULTIPLE CHOICE

18. Which of the following statements does *not* refer to vitamin B$_{12}$ (cyanocobalamin)?

    a. Important in cell replication

    b. Lack of results in pernicious anemia

    c. Important in myelin synthesis

    d. Deficiency results in uremia

19. Patient education related to vitamins must include which of the following statements?

    a. Specific reason for prescribed vitamin therapy

    b. Monitoring specific brands being taken by the patient

    c. RDAs as stated on the label

    d. Only low-income groups suffer from deficiencies

20. Which of the following vitamins would you recommend for tissue healing?

    a. Vitamin D (ergocalciferol)

    b. Vitamin E (tocopherols)

    c. Vitamin A (Aquasol)

    d. Vitamin C (ascorbic acid)

21. Enteral nutrition includes all of the following routes except which one?

    a. Intravenous tube feeding

    b. Nasogastric tube feeding

    c. Gastrostomy tube feeding

    d. Oral feeding

22. Your patient is likely to receive total parenteral nutrition (TPN) for which of the following conditions?

    a. Major surgery

    b. Bowel obstruction

    c. Supplement oral intake

    d. Difficulty swallowing

23. Macrominerals or microminerals require patient education of which of the following?

    a. They should be taken at less than the recommended RDA.

    b. They are organic substances necessary to maintain homeostasis.

    c. All can reach toxic levels unless taken as prescribed.

    d. Minerals are necessary for lipid lowering to occur.

24. Patient education for TPN must include which of the following?

    a. Clean technique when changing dressings and tubings

    b. Signs and symptoms of hyperglycemia

    c. Need to report increased feelings of hunger

    d. Stabilization of nutritional status

25. When the patient is on loop diuretics, the nurse will need to assess which of the following?

    a. Potassium level

    b. Sodium level

    c. Magnesium level

    d. All of the above

26. Hypomagnesemia will produce which of the following symptoms?

    a. Nausea, vomiting, and constipation

    b. Weakness, anorexia, and bleeding abnormalities

    c. Muscular twitches, cramps, and spasms

    d. General weakness, hypertension, and respiratory depression

27. Why must patients receiving TPN be monitored for fluid volume excess/overload?

    a. TPN is a hypertonic solution that can cause a fluid shift.

    b. Endogenous insulin is insufficient for glucose metabolism.

    c. Strict aseptic technique will prevent infections.

    d. Weighing will assist with monitoring intake and output.

MAKING CONNECTIONS

28. Your patient complains of gnawing pain in the epigastric area that is temporarily relieved by food, but then recurs within 30 min after eating. With a history of PUD, which diagnosis should be suspected?

    a. Gastric ulcer

    b. Duodenal ulcer

    c. Crohn's disease

    d. IBS

29. Diphenoxylate with atropine (Lomotil) is an opioid that is given to relieve diarrhea. Why is atropine added to this medication?

    a. To prevent abuse of this medication

    b. To dry up loose stools and secretions

    c. To provide an anticholinergic response

    d. To provide a cholinergic response

30. Psyllium mucilloid (Metamucil) is a bulk former that is used with which of the following combinations?

    a. Laxative or anti-diarrheal

    b. Laxative or anti-emetic

    c. Anti-diarrheal or anti-flatulent

    d. Anti-diarrheal or anti-emetic

31. Scopolamine (Transderm-Scop) is an effective anti-emetic that is usually prescribed as which of the following?

    a. Liquid suspension

    b. Subcutaneous injection

    c. Dermal patch

    d. Intramuscular injection

32. Herbal remedies for diarrhea include which of the following preparations?

    a. Senna root

    b. Cascara leaves

    c. Acidophilus

    d. Sibutramine

CALCULATIONS

33. The patient has pernicious anemia. The order reads: Administer cyanocobalamin 200 mcg/month IM. The vial reads 100 mcg/ml in a 30 ml vial. How much will the nurse give per monthly dose?

34. The patient has hypomagnesemia. He is about to receive 250 mg in 250 ml over 4 hours. How many milliliters per hour will he receive?

CASE STUDY APPLICATIONS

35. Mr. W, age 78, has developed aspiration pneumonia due to an impaired swallowing reflex. The physician has decided to place a gastroscopy tube for enteral feedings. He is to be placed on a specialized feeding. During your initial assessment, you determine the following:

    a. Because of his respiratory condition, he will require a custom food supplement. Which would you recommend? Why?

    b. Laboratory tests will determine his ability to heal. What laboratory results will you need to monitor?

    c. Name the four types of enteral feedings that are available.

    d. What is your overall goal for this patient?

    e. What nursing interventions will you employ to aid in achieving this goal?

    f. What evaluative criteria will you use to determine if the goal was met?

36. Mrs. G has a stroke, so the nurse believes that TPN is in order. Your patient goes to the OR for the insertion of a central line. During your post-op assessment you note the solution infusing at the site of insertion.

    a. What type of solution will this patient receive?

    b. Why is this form of feeding necessary?

    c. What is the short-term goal for this patient?

    d. What is the long-term goal for this patient?

    e. What nursing interventions are required in this patient's care?

    f. How will you evaluate the effectiveness of the plan of care?

37. Mr. S is admitted with malabsorption syndrome secondary to chemotherapy. The doctor discusses with him the need for central line placement for this procedure.

    a. Why is a central line necessary? What NANDA diagnosis would you use for this patient?

    b. Will this type of feeding be short term? What is your goal for this patient?

    c. Can the patient return home with this type of feeding?

CHAPTER 39

DRUGS FOR PITUITARY, THYROID, AND ADRENAL DISORDERS

OBJECTIVES

To view the objectives, please refer to the textbook, student CD-ROM, and the Companion Website at *www.prenhall.com/adams*.

FILL IN THE BLANK

From the textbook, find the correct word(s) to complete the statements(s).

1. _____ are chemical messengers released in response to a change in the body's internal environment.

2. Releasing hormones signal the _____ to release the hormone necessary to create a desired effect in the body.

3. When administering antidiuretic hormones, the nurse should carefully assess fluid and _____ balance.

4. Vasopressin injection (Pitressin) should never be administered by the _____ route.

5. Prior to administration of levothyroxine (Synthroid), the nurse should thoroughly assess the patient's _____ system.

6. Graves' disease may cause tachycardia, weight loss, elevated body temperature, and _____.

7. Propylthiouracil (PTU) may cause GI distress and should be administered _____ meals.

8. The nurse must be aware that glucocorticoids increase the patient's susceptibility to _____.

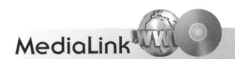

MediaLink

www.prenhall.com/adams

CD-ROM
Audio Glossary
NCLEX Review

Companion Website
NCLEX Review
Dosage Calculations
Case Study
Care Plans
Expanded Key Concepts

MATCHING

For questions 9 through 13, match the specific disease in column I with its related concept in column II.

Column I	Column II
9. _____ Cushing's syndrome	a. Thyroid hormone (Synthroid)
10. _____ Adrenal cortex hyposecretion	b. Vasopressin (Pitressin)
11. _____ Graves' disease	c. Linked to glucocorticoid use
12. _____ Myxedema (adults) and cretinism (children)	d. Glucocorticoids
13. _____ Diabetes insipidus	e. Propylthiouracil (PTU)

For questions 14 through 16, match the drug in column I with its class in column II.

Column I	Column II
14. _____ Prednisone (Deltasone, others)	a. Thyroid medication
15. _____ Liotrix (Euthroid, others)	b. Antithyroid medication
16. _____ Methimazole (Tapazole)	c. Glucocorticoid

MULTIPLE CHOICE

17. The nurse is monitoring a patient's lab tests and notices a rise in parathyroid hormone (PTH). Which of the following lab values may also occur in this patient?

    a. Increased blood glucose

    b. Decreased blood glucose

    c. Decreased serum calcium

    d. Increased serum calcium

18. The nurse understands that negative feedback ensures endocrine homeostasis by doing which of the following?

    a. Stimulating the release of a secondary hormone

    b. Stimulating the release of a primary hormone

    c. Inhibiting the action of a secondary hormone

    d. Inhibiting the action of a primary hormone

19. The nurse is caring for a patient who is receiving hormone replacement therapy (HRT). Which of the following is *not* an example of HRT?

    a. Thyroid hormone after thyroidectomy

    b. Supplying insulin to a patient whose pancreas is not functioning

    c. Testosterone for breast cancer

    d. Adrenal cortex dysfunction

20. Which of the following hormones is *not* released from the anterior pituitary gland?

    a. Thyroid-stimulating hormone (TSH)

    b. Antidiuretic hormone

    c. Growth hormone

    d. Adrenocorticotropic hormone (ACTH)

21. A patient receiving levothyroxine (Synthroid) may experience which of the following adverse effects?

    a. Loss of weight

    b. Lack of energy

    c. Reduced pulse rate

    d. Reduced body temperature

22. It is important that the nurse teach female patients that long-term use of levothyroxine (Synthroid) may be associated with which of the following symptoms?

    a. Osteoporosis

    b. Decreased white blood cell count

    c. Weight gain

    d. Decreased incidence of insomnia

23. The nurse would most likely administer antithyroid medications to patients with which of the following symptoms?

    a. Dysrhythmia

    b. Weight loss

    c. Reduced activity

    d. Anemia

24. Which of the following hormones will ultimately result in release of glucocorticoids from the adrenal glands?

    a. Corticotropin releasing factor (CRF)

    b. Adrenocorticotropic hormone (ACTH)

    c. Falling levels of cortisol

    d. All of the above

25. Which of the following drugs is often administered by alternate-day dosing and requires the nurse to provide specific patient teaching?

    a. Thyroid hormone

    b. Antithyroid therapy

    c. Corticosteroids

    d. Insulin

26. In caring for a patient with Cushing's syndrome, the nurse understands this disorder is associated with which of the following hormones?

    a. Mineralocorticoids

    b. Glucocorticoids

    c. Androgens

    d. ADH

27. The nurse should observe for which of the following adverse effects of hydrocortisone (Cortef, Hydrocortone) therapy?

    a. Asthma

    b. Rhinitis

    c. Nausea

    d. Mood and personality changes

28. Which of the following corticosteroids has mineralocorticoid activity?

    a. Hydrocortisone (Cortef, Hydrocortone)

    b. Methylprednisolone (Solu-Medrol, Medrol)

    c. Prednisolone (Delta-Cortef)

    d. Prednisone (Deltasone, others)

29. A deficiency of growth hormone will result in which of the following?

    a. Dwarfism

    b. Diabetes insipidus

    c. Urinary retention

    d. Mental impairment

30. Vasopressin (Pitressin) is prescribed for which of the following primary symptoms?

    a. Altered metabolism

    b. Polyuria

    c. Inflammation

    d. Altered glucose blood levels

MAKING CONNECTIONS

31. Which of the following will change during thyroid therapy if only heart rate increases?

    a. Dysrhythmia

    b. Peripheral vascular resistance

    c. Cardiac output

    d. Stroke volume

32. Cholestyramine (Questran) will decrease the absorption of levothyroxine (Synthroid) if given at the same time. Patients take cholestyramine for what type of disorders?

    a. Hypertension

    b. High blood cholesterol levels

    c. Peptic ulcers

    d. Weight gain

33. Fluconazole (Diflucan) and other azole drugs are indicated for which of the following?

    a. Fungal infections

    b. Malaria

    c. Diarrhea

    d. Constipation

34. Which vitamin is considered to be an antidote for overdoses of warfarin (Coumadin)?

    a. A

    b. B_2

    c. B_{12}

    d. K

35. A drug's trade name is assigned by which of the following?

    a. Physician

    b. Pharmacist

    c. Drug manufacturer

    d. FDA

CALCULATIONS

36. The physician ordered Pitressin 10 U SC bid for a patient. The pharmacy has Pitressin 20 U/ml. How many milliliters will the nurse administer?

37. The physician ordered propylthiouracil 200 mg PO for a patient. The pharmacy has propylthiouracil 50 mg tablets. How many tablets will the nurse administer?

CASE STUDY APPLICATIONS

38. Ms. Z is diabetic and is also a candidate for thyroid therapy because of her hypothyroid disorder. Examples of the medications she might take include levothyroxine sodium (Synthroid, others), liothyronine sodium (Cytomel), and liotrix (Euthroid, others).

    a. In planning proper care, what complications of using these drugs simultaneously would the nurse consider?

    b. What nursing interventions would be appropriate?

39. Mr. D, age 35, is diagnosed with Graves' disease. He wants to know how his new medication propylthiouracil (PTU) will impact his life.

    a. List the important patient teaching related to PTU.

    b. Describe nursing interventions that will assist this patient in adjusting to his medication regimen.

CHAPTER 40

DRUGS FOR PANCREATIC DISORDERS

OBJECTIVES

To view the objectives, please refer to the textbook, student CD-ROM, and the Companion Website at *www.prenhall.com/adams*.

FILL IN THE BLANK

From the textbook, find the correct word(s) to complete the statements(s).

1. Juvenile-onset diabetes is called _____; age-onset

   diabetes is referred to as _____.

2. A class of drugs prescribed after diet and exercise have failed to bring blood glucose levels to within normal limits is

   _____.

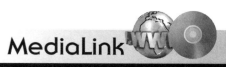

MediaLink

www.prenhall.com/adams

CD-ROM
Animation:
   Mechanism in Action: Glipizide
   (Glucotrol)
Audio Glossary
NCLEX Review

Companion Website
NCLEX Review
Dosage Calculations
Case Study
Care Plans
Expanded Key Concepts

3. In type 2 diabetes mellitus, insulin receptors in the target tissues have become _____ to the hormone.

4. The treatment goal with insulin therapy is to maintain _____ levels within strict, normal limits.

5. Acute pancreatitis may occur suddenly and most commonly exhibits symptoms of _____.

6. _____ elevates the protein content of pancreatic juices, and contributes to the formation of stones which may block pancreatic ducts.

MATCHING

For questions 7 through 9, match the specific disease in column I with the drug therapy in column II.

Column I	Column II
7. _____ Type I diabetes mellitus	a. Pancrelipase (Lipancreatin)
8. _____ Type II diabetes mellitus	b. Regular insulin (Humulin R)

9. _____ Chronic pancreatitis

c. Glipizide (Glucotrol)

For questions 10 through 12, match the drug in column I with its class in column II.

Column I	Column II
10. _____ Pancrelipase (Lipancreatin)	a. Hypoglycemics
11. _____ Regular insulin (Humulin R)	b. Insulin
12. _____ Glipizide (Glucotrol)	c. Pancreatic enzyme replacement

MULTIPLE CHOICE

13. Which of the following stimulates the pancreas to secrete insulin?

   a. Hyperglycemia

   b. Hypoglycemia

   c. Glucagon

   d. Ketoacids

14. While taking a health history, the nurse should recognize that which of the following is *not* a short-term sign of type 1 diabetes mellitus?

   a. Polyuria

   b. Polyphagia

   c. Acidosis

   d. Polydipsia

15. When giving insulin, the nurse knows the most common route of administration is which of the following?

   a. Oral

   b. Intradermal

   c. Subcutaneous

   d. Intramuscular

16. When planning follow-up care, the nurse should know that which of the following is a longer-acting form of insulin?

   a. Insulin lispro (Humalog)

   b. Insulin, isophane (Humulin N, others)

   c. Insulin lente (Humulin L, Novolin L, others)

   d. Insulin ultralente (Humulin U, Ultralente)

17. Which of the following adverse effects does the nurse recognize when too much insulin has been administered?

   a. Hypoglycemia

   b. Tachycardia

   c. Convulsions

   d. All of the above

18. When giving oral hypoglycemics, the nurse expects which of the following actions to occur?

    a. The pancreas is stimulated to secrete more insulin.

    b. Insulin receptors become more sensitive to target tissues.

    c. The liver is inhibited from releasing glucose.

    d. Both a and b

19. Which of the following administration techniques applies to pancrelipase (Ultrase)?

    a. Crush enteric-coated tablets.

    b. Swallow enteric-coated tablets.

    c. Give 4 hours following meals.

    d. Give slow IV push.

20. During oral hypoglycemic therapy, the nurse should assess for which symptoms related to abnormalities in liver function?

    a. Yellowed skin, pale stools, dark urine

    b. Pink skin, light brown stools, yellow urine

    c. Pale skin, red-tinged stools, amber urine

    d. Red skin, dark stools, clear urine

21. If injections sites are not rotated regularly, the diabetic patient may suffer from which of the following?

    a. Petechiae

    b. Lipodystrophy

    c. Hematoma

    d. Pustules

22. Which of the following nursing diagnoses is *not* appropriate for the patient receiving insulin therapy?

    a. Risk for injury

    b. Risk for imbalanced nutrition

    c. Risk for role confusion

    d. Risk for infection

23. When considering glucose regulation in the body, which of the following components of homeostasis would be restored following insulin therapy?

    a. Sensor (senses glucose in the bloodstream)

    b. Control center (determines the set point for glucose levels in the bloodstream)

    c. Effector (responds to the increased levels of glucose in the bloodstream)

    d. Receptor (produces a response at the site of glucose action)

MAKING CONNECTIONS

24. A patient is prescribed pancrelipase (Ultrase), and also takes iron supplements. The nurse is aware that taking these drugs together may do which of the following?

    a. Increase iron absorption

    b. Decrease iron absorption

    c. Increase zymase absorption

    d. Decrease zymase absorption

25. Prior to administration of medications for pancreatitis, the nurse understands that assessing for alcohol abuse is necessary because alcohol can do which of the following?

    a. Contribute to stone formation and pancreatic inflammation

    b. Cause inhibition of gastric secretions

    c. Enhance lung expansion

    d. Elevate blood pH

26. Why must the nurse instruct a patient receiving glipizide (Glucotrol XL) to avoid crushing or chewing the tablets?

    a. The patient may choke.

    b. The effectiveness of the medication would be hindered.

    c. It would cause blood glucose levels to rise too rapidly.

    d. Irritation of the oral mucosa may occur.

27. MAO inhibitors may potentiate hypoglycemic effects when used with which of the following drugs?

    a. Insulin

    b. Dextrothyroxine

    c. Corticosteroids

    d. Epinephrine

CALCULATIONS

28. The physician ordered Humulin L lente U100 35 U SC, regular Humulin R U100 20 U. A U-/100 insulin syringe is available. What is the total amount of insulin to be given?

29. The physician ordered glipizide 10 mg PO daily. The pharmacy has glipizide 5 mg. How many tablets will the nurse administer?

CASE STUDY APPLICATIONS

30. Mr. D is 70 years old and has diabetes mellitus type 2. You are performing an initial assessment.

    a. In planning Mr. D's nursing care, which kind of diabetic therapy would he likely require?

    b. Explain the patient teaching needed for Mr. D, including difficulties that may arise.

31. The nurse is planning discharge teaching for Mr. C, a patient recently diagnosed with chronic pancreatitis. He lives alone, has little to no income, and does not have transportation.

    a. What important points should the nurse include in her discharge planning?

    b. What data from patient's social history will take special analysis when planning care?

CHAPTER 41

DRUGS FOR DISORDERS AND CONDITIONS OF THE FEMALE REPRODUCTIVE SYSTEM

OBJECTIVES

To view the objectives, please refer to the textbook, student CD-ROM, and the Companion Website at *www.prenhall.com/adams*.

FILL IN THE BLANK

From the textbook, find the correct word(s) to complete the statements(s).

1. _____ is the hormone that regulates sperm or egg

   production; _____ in the female triggers the release
   of the egg, a process known as ovulation.

2. The permanent cessation of menses, caused by lack of estrogen

   secretion by the ovaries, is _____.

3. A class of drugs called _____ exerts positive metabolic effects in postmenopausal women including
   an increase in bone mass and a reduction in LDL cholesterol.

4. The absence of menstruation is called _____.

5. A class of drugs called _____ is often prescribed for dysfunctional uterine bleeding.

6. The anterior pituitary hormone _____ increases the synthesis of milk within the mammary glands;

   the posterior pituitary hormone _____ causes milk to be ejected.

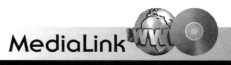

MediaLink

www.prenhall.com/adams

CD-ROM
Animation:
   Mechanism in Action: Ortho-Novum
Audio Glossary
NCLEX Review

Companion Website
NCLEX Review
Dosage Calculations
Case Study
Care Plans
Expanded Key Concepts

MATCHING

For questions 7 through 10, match the drug in column I with its classification in column II.

Column I	Column II
7. _____ Norethindrone (Micronor)	a. Estrogens
8. _____ Terbutaline sulfate (Brethine)	b. Uterine stimulants
9. _____ Misoprostol (Cytotec)	c. Tocolytics
10. _____ Estradiol valerate (Delestrogen, others)	d. Progestin

For questions 11 through 15, match the drug classification in column I with its indication in column II. Use each answer only once.

Column I	Column II
11. _____ Progestins	a. To prevent conception
12. _____ Estrogens	b. Dysfunctional uterine bleeding
13. _____ Oral contraceptives	c. Replacement therapy in women and prostate cancer in men
14. _____ Oxytocin	d. Premature labor
15. _____ Tocolytics	e. To induce labor

MULTIPLE CHOICE

16. The nurse is to administer a triphasic type of oral contraceptive. Which of the following is classified in this manner?

    a. Alesse

    b. Lo/Ovral

    c. Ortho-Cyclin

    d. Ortho-Novum

17. Which of the following potential consequences of estrogen loss related to postmenopausal conditions should be included in a teaching plan for the postmenopausal patient?

    a. Insomnia

    b. Sexual disinterest

    c. Mood disturbances

    d. Osteoporosis

18. Which of the following drugs is used to treat endometriosis is a GnRH agonist?

    a. Estropipate (Ogen)

    b. Ethinyl estradiol (Ethinyl, Feminone)

    c. Estradiol (Estraderm, Estrace)

    d. Leuprolide (Lupron)

19. The nurse understands that which of the following uterine stimulants may also be used for short-term treatment of gastric ulcers?

    a. Oxytocin (Pitocin, Syntocinon)

    b. Misoprostol (Cytotec)

    c. Dinoprostone (Cervidil, others)

    d. Methylergonovine maleate (Methergine)

20. The following medications may be prescribed for the patient with preeclampsia. The nurse understands which of these may also be used as an anticonvulsant?

    a. Oxytocin (Pitocin)

    b. Magnesium sulfate

    c. Terbutaline sulfate (Brethine)

    d. Ritodrine hydrochloride (Yutopar)

21. In developing a teaching plan for the patient taking oral contraceptives, the nurse teaches which of the following may decrease the effectiveness of her chosen method of contraception?

    a. Antibiotics

    b. Antineoplastics

    c. Calcium channel blockers

    d. Antihypertensives

22. Which endocrine gland(s) releases steroid hormones such as estrogen and androgens?

    a. Pituitary gland

    b. Pancreas

    c. Adrenal glands

    d. Hypothalamus

23. The nurse teaches her patient that the oral contraceptive she is taking is effective because it produces a thick cervical mucus. Which of the following medications has this action?

    a. Progesterone micronized (Prometrium)

    b. Estradiol (Estraderm, Estrace)

    c. Danazol (Danocrine)

    d. Nandrolone phenpropionate (Durabolin, Hybolin)

24. Which of the following drugs is used for termination of early pregnancy?

    a. Estropipate (Ogen)

    b. Fluoxymesterone (Halotestin)

    c. Mifepristone (RU 486)

    d. Ritodrine hydrochloride (Yutopar)

25. Which of the following would *not* be included in the teaching plan as a benefit of conjugated estrogen and progestin therapy?

    a. Lowered risk of colon cancer

   b. Reduction in LDL cholesterol

   c. Weight loss

   d. Increase in bone mass

26. The school nurse teaches a group of 9-year-old girls that the function of natural progesterone is which of the following?

   a. To build up the lining of the uterus

   b. To prevent ovulation

   c. To prepare the uterus for implantation of the embryo

   d. To begin the onset of menstrual bleeding

27. The nurse is screening a patient for the appropriateness of oral contraceptive use. He understands that oral contraceptives are contraindicated in patients with which of the following disorders?

   a. Hypertension

   b. Hyperglycemia

   c. Potential for blood clots and stroke

   d. Depression

MAKING CONNECTIONS

28. Relating to women's healthcare, where would barbiturate thiopental sodium (Pentothal) most likely be used?

   a. Coronary care unit

   b. Sleep disorder clinic

   c. Cancer clinic

   d. Surgical suite

29. What is the classification of interferon alpha-2a?

   a. Alkylating agent

   b. Biologic response modifier

   c. Hormone

   d. Coagulation modifier

30. Which of the following drugs, if given in high doses, could induce hypothyroidism?

   a. Amiodarone (Cordarone)

   b. Finasteride (Proscar)

   c. Repaglinide (Prandin)

   d. Rosiglitazone (Avandia)

31. A diabetic patient is also diagnosed with hypothyroidism. Which of the following reactions to treatment with levothyroxine (Synthroid) would be most expected?

    a. Immediate improvement of symptoms

    b. Initial worsening of symptoms

    c. No change in symptoms

    d. Decreased need for insulin

32. A diabetic patient asks about using Stevia as a sugar substitute. Which of the following is *not* true about Stevia?

    a. It is an herb found in Paraguay.

    b. It sweetens foods better than sugar.

    c. It is approved by the FDA.

    d. It does not appear to have a negative effect on blood glucose.

CALCULATIONS

33. The physician ordered gonadorelin (Factrel) 100 mcg IVPB added to 100 cc D5W to be infused over 2 hours. The drop factor is 15 gtt/cc How many gtt/min should be given to infuse the total amount in 2 hours?

34. The physician ordered Depo-Provera 100 mg IM. The pharmacy has 400 mg/ml. How many milliliters will the nurse administer?

CASE STUDY APPLICATIONS

35. Ms. M, at age 50, is concerned about the unpleasant effects accompanying menopause. Her last menstrual period was several months ago, and she is beginning to experience hot flashes, night sweats, nervousness, and insomnia. The nurse suggests hormone replacement therapy (HRT). Ms. M states she knows nothing about HRT.

    a. What nursing diagnosis is appropriate for Ms. M? State the expected outcome for this nursing diagnosis.

    b. State the patient teaching necessary to assist Ms. M in achieving the expected outcome.

36. Mrs. E, a primigravida who is 30 weeks pregnant, is in labor. Following rupture of membranes she is receiving oxytocin IV.

    a. What assessment data are necessary for the nurse to gather to monitor for adverse effects?

    b. List nursing actions related to this medication.

CHAPTER 42

DRUGS FOR DISORDERS AND CONDITIONS OF THE MALE REPRODUCTIVE SYSTEM

OBJECTIVES

To view the objectives, please refer to the textbook, student CD-ROM, and the Companion Website at *www.prenhall.com/adams*.

FILL IN THE BLANK

From the textbook, find the correct word(s) to complete the statements(s).

1. _____ are testosterone-like compounds with hormonal activity.

2. A side effect of testosterone therapy in female patients is the appearance of masculine characteristics

   or _____.

3. The oral medication first approved for erectile dysfunction in 1998 was _____.

4. _____ is an enlargement of the prostate gland that occurs mostly in men of advanced age.

5. _____ are sex hormones found in male and female patients.

6. Testosterone (Andro) is a category _____ drug and should not be taken if pregnancy is suspected or confirmed.

7. _____ have been approved to treat benign enlargement of the prostate.

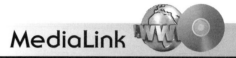

MATCHING

For questions 8 through12, match the drug in column I with its classification in column II.

Column I	Column II
8. _____ Testosterone base (Andro LA)	a. Androgens
9. _____ Prazosin (Minipress)	b. Alpha-adrenergic blocker
10. _____ Finasteride (Proscar)	c. Alpha-reductase inhibitor
11. _____ Danazol (Danocrine)	
12. _____ Terazosin (Hytrin)	

MULTIPLE CHOICE

13. The patient is concerned about erectile dysfunction. The nurse understands that this condition may be successfully treated with which of the following?

    a. Testosterone (Andro 100, others)

    b. Sildenafil (Viagra)

    c. Finasteride (Proscar)

    d. Doxazosin (Cardura)

14. When screening for risk factors for erectile dysfunction, the nurse should ask the patient about which of the following diseases?

    a. Diabetes

    b. Hypertension

    c. Benign prostatic hyperplasia (BPH)

    d. Both a and b

15. The nurse must include which of the following adverse effects when providing teaching to a patient receiving anabolic steroids?

    a. Liver damage

    b. Appearance of masculine characteristics

    c. Muscle weakness

    d. Cardiovascular disease

16. The nurse recognizes the patient is taking a natural therapy for BPH when the patient states he is taking which of the following?

    a. Saw palmetto

    b. Ginkgo biloba

    c. St. John's wort

    d. Black cohosh

17. Androgens may be abused by which of the following?

    a. Older adults to improve sexual function

    b. Athletes to improve athletic performance

   c. College students to increase mental acuity

   d. Middle-aged men to arrest hair loss

18. The nurse recognizes which of the following as a symptom of male hypogonadism?

   a. Abundant axillary hair

   b. Decrease in subcutaneous fat

   c. Reduced libido

   d. Hyperactivity

19. The wife of a patient taking anabolic steroids reports to the nurse that her husband has become aggressive. What is the most appropriate response?

   a. "Try speaking to your husband in a low, calm voice."

   b. "Tell me about your behavior prior to his aggressive acts."

   c. "Have you contacted the domestic abuse hotline?"

   d. "This is a common behavioral change related to anabolic steroid use."

20. Instructions for applying a testosterone transdermal patch would include to change sites how frequently?

   a. q72h and rotate sites every 3 days

   b. q2h and rotate sites every 14 days

   c. q24h and rotate sites every 7 days

   d. q4h and rotate sites every 10 days

21. The nurse must routinely monitor which of the following lab values for a patient receiving androgen therapy?

   a. Serum cholesterol

   b. Hematocrit

   c. Prothrombin time

   d. Alpha fetoprotein

22. The nurse understands which of the following drugs to be contraindicated when used concurrently with sildenafil (Viagra)?

   a. Nitroglycerin

   b. Sulfonamides

   c. Sodium bicarbonate

   d. Reglan

23. Which of the following nurses should not be assigned to administer medication to the patient receiving finasteride (Proscar)?

   a. Mike, age 29, LPN with male pattern baldness

   b. Lydia, age 35, registered nurse with a cold

   c. Jack, age 40, recently licensed practical nurse

   d. Susan, age 25, pregnant registered nurse

MAKING CONNECTIONS

24. Stress often has an effect on the release of hormones. Which of the following nervous system components would activate hormonal release at the level of the hypothalamus and adrenal glands?

    a. Somatic nervous system

    b. Sympathetic nervous system

    c. Central nervous system

    d. Sensory nervous system

25. Glucocorticoids would produce an effect at which of the following target receptor locations?

    a. Plasma membrane of the target cell

    b. Cytoplasm of the target cell

    c. Nucleus of the target cell

    d. Cellular component other than the nucleus

26. Cimetidine (Tagamet) is sometimes given to patients who are taking glucocorticoids in order to prevent which disorder?

    a. Hypertension

    b. Constipation

    c. Thromboembolic disease

    d. Peptic ulcer disease

27. The nurse understands an adolescent diabetic's therapeutic regime is compromised when he states which of the following?

    a. "I'll eat ice cream at the party and take more insulin."

    b. "Taking my blood sugar at the party will be uncomfortable."

    c. "I'll bring my insulin and syringes to the party."

    d. "I can eat party foods that contain protein."

28. In teaching a diabetic patient how to control his blood glucose, the nurse should encourage him to keep the preprandial blood glucose level at which level?

    a. Below 50 mg/dl

    b. Below 110 mg/dl

    c. Above 50 mg/dl

    d. Above 110 mg/dl

CALCULATIONS

29. The physician ordered danazol (Danocrine) 150 mg PO. The pharmacy has 100 mg tablets. How many tablets will the nurse administer?

30. The physician ordered terazosin (Hytrin) 4 mg PO. The pharmacy has 2 mg capsules. How many capsules will the nurse administer?

CASE STUDY APPLICATIONS

31. Mr. E, a 62-year-old patient, is receiving finasteride (Proscar) due to an enlarged prostate. He asks the nurse how he will know if the medication is working and when he can stop taking it.

    a. List the nursing interventions and patient teaching appropriate for Mr. E.

    b. State specifically how the nurse will evaluate medication effectiveness.

32. Mr. S, a 38-year-old married man, has been diagnosed with low testosterone levels. Mr. S is a type 1 diabetic and prides himself in his knowledge of herb use related to health.

    a. What assessment data are important for the nurse to obtain before Mr. S begins androgen therapy?

    b. What nursing interventions and patient education are appropriate for Mr. S related to his diabetes?

CHAPTER 43

DRUGS FOR RENAL DISORDERS AND DIURETIC THERAPY

OBJECTIVES

To view the objectives, please refer to the textbook, student CD-ROM, and the Companion Website at *www.prenhall.com/adams*.

FILL IN THE BLANK

From the textbook, find the correct word(s) to complete the statements(s).

1. Thiazide diuretics act on the _____ tubule of the nephron.

2. Sodium and potassium are exchanged in the _____ tubule, where Na$^+$ is _____ back into the body and K$^+$ is _____ into the tubule.

3. Each kidney contains over a million _____, the functional units of the kidney.

4. Identify the parts of the nephron shown in Figure 43–1.

   A. _____

   B. _____

   C. _____

   D. _____

   E. _____

   F. _____

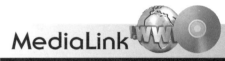

MediaLink

www.prehnall.com/adams

CD-ROM
Animation:
  Basic Function of the Kidney
Audio Glossary
NCLEX Review

Companion Website
NCLEX Review
Dosage Calculations
Case Study
Care Plans

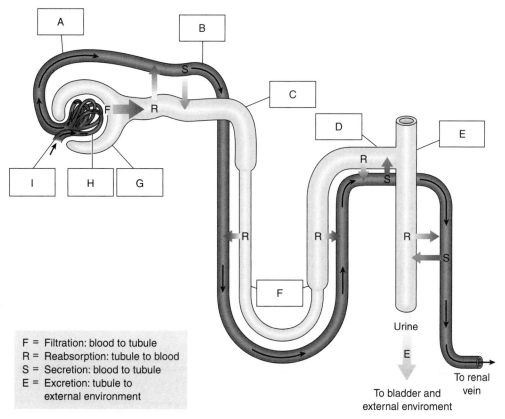

Figure 43–1

SOURCE: Core Concepts in Pharmacology, Workbook by Holland/Adams, © 2003. Reprinted by permission of Pearson Education, Inc., Upper Saddle River, NJ.

G. _____

H. _____

I. _____

MATCHING

For questions 5 through 16, match the drug in column I with its classification in column II.

Column I	Column II
5. _____ Bumetanide (Bumex)	a. Loop diuretic
6. _____ Benzthiazide (Aquatag, Exna, Hydrex)	b. Thiazide or thiazide-like diuretic
7. _____ Triamterene (Dyrenium)	c. Potassium-sparing diuretic
8. _____ Metolazone (Zaroxolyn, Mykrox)	d. Carbonic anhydrase inhibitor diuretic
9. _____ Mannitol (Osmitrol)	e. Osmotic diuretic
10. _____ Quinethazone (Hydromox)	
11. _____ Spironolactone (Aldactone)	
12. _____ Acetazolamide (Diamox)	

13. _____ Furosemide (Lasix)

14. _____ Methazolamide (Neptazane)

15. _____ Hydrochlorothiazide (HydroDIURIL, HCTZ)

16. _____ Indapamide (Lozol)

MULTIPLE CHOICE

17. The nurse administering medications understands that reabsorption and secretion are critical to pharmacokinetics. The composition of the filtrate that passes through Bowman's capsule is similar to which of the following?

    a. Plasma

    b. Plasma minus large proteins

    c. Urine

    d. Blood

18. Medications in the filtrate that pass across the walls of the nephron to reenter the blood use what process?

    a. Reabsorption

    b. Urination

    c. Secretion

    d. Absorption

19. Drugs, such as penicillin G, which are too large to pass through Bowman's capsule, enter the urine by crossing from the blood to the filtrate using what process?

    a. Excretion

    b. Reabsorption

    c. Metabolism

    d. Secretion

20. The nurse explains to the patient that the main function of a diuretic is to increase which of the following?

    a. Reabsorption of water in the nephron

    b. Blood flow through Bowman's capsule

    c. Urine output

    d. Secretion of water in the nephron

21. The nurse understands that most diuretics act by blocking the reabsorption in the nephron of which of the following?

    a. Large proteins

    b. Potassium

    c. Electrolytes

    d. Sodium

22. Which of the following classes of diuretics can cause large amounts of fluid to be excreted by the kidney in a short time when administered IV?

    a. Loop

    b. Thiazides

    c. Osmotic

    d. Potassium-sparing

23. Medications that block reabsorption of sodium also affect the amount of water in the filtrate. What effect (if any) does this have on urine flow?

    a. No effect

    b. Increased flow

    c. Decreased flow

    d. Flow may increase or decrease depending on lifestyle factors

24. Which of the following is a relatively common and serious side effect of diuretic therapy?

    a. Edema

    b. Hyperkalemia

    c. Dehydration

    d. Hypertension

25. The nurse must monitor for which of the following adverse effects specific to the loop class of diuretics?

    a. Hepatotoxicity

    b. Ototoxicity

    c. Dehydration

    d. Acidosis

26. Which of the following is the most widely prescribed class of diuretics?

    a. Loop/high-ceiling diuretics

    b. Potassium sparing

    c. Carbonic anhydrase inhibitors

    d. Thiazides

27. Which patient is most likely to be administered thiazide diuretics?

    a. 50-year-old male with mild to moderate hypertension

    b. 34-year-old female with pyelonephritis

    c. 80-year-old with dehydration

    d. 60-year-old with lung cancer

28. The nurse teaches the patient that intake of potassium-rich foods should *not* be increased during therapy with which of the following medications?

    a. Furosemide (Lasix)

    b. Chlorothiazide (Diuril)

    c. Spironolactone (Aldactone)

    d. Acetazolamide (Diamox)

29. Spironolactone (Aldactone) acts by inhibiting which of the following?

    a. Aldosterone

    b. Carbonic anhydrase

    c. Potassium reabsorption in the distal tubule

    d. Sodium reabsorption in the loop of Henle

30. Which diuretic is prescribed specifically to decrease intraocular fluid pressure in patients with open-angle glaucoma?

    a. Torsemide (Demadex)

    b. Triamterene (Dyrenium)

    c. Chlorthalidone (Hygroton)

    d. Acetazolamide (Diamox)

MAKING CONNECTIONS

31. Indapamide (Lozol) is a thiazide-like diuretic that is chemically related to sulfonamides. What are many sulfonamides used to treat?

    a. Peptic ulcers

    b. Viral infections

    c. Bacterial infections

    d. Anxiety

32. Scopolamine (Transderm-Scop) is an anticholinergic drug primarily used for which of the following?

    a. Dysrhythmias

    b. Hypertension

    c. Inflammation

    d. Motion sickness

33. Dyphylline (Dilor) is a xanthine drug similar to theophylline; it relaxes smooth muscle. What is its primary indication?

    a. Shock

    b. Asthma

    c. Parkinson's disease

    d. Migraines

34. A female patient is prescribed nafarelin (Synarel) inhalant. Which of the following administration instructions is it important for the nurse to give?

    a. One inhalation beginning between day 5 and 10 of menstrual cycle

    b. Two inhalations beginning between day 2 and 5 of menstrual cycle

    c. One inhalation beginning between day 2 and 4 of menstrual cycle

    d. Two inhalations beginning between day 5 and 10 of menstrual cycle

35. All of the following affect circadian rhythm and therefore the medication regimen except which one?

    a. Temperature

    b. Hour of sleep

    c. Blood pressure

    d. Age at menarche

CALCULATIONS

36. The physician ordered metolazone (Mykrox) 1 mg PO. The pharmacy has 0.5 mg tablets. How many tablets will the nurse administer?

37. The physician ordered acetazolamide (Diamox) 500 mg IVPB added to 100 cc D5W to be infused over 2 hours. The drop factor is 10 gtt/cc. How many gtt/min should be given to infuse the total amount in 2 hours?

CASE STUDY APPLICATIONS

38. Mr. S is an active 56-year-old who was diagnosed with hypertension 12 months ago. At that time, he was placed on verapamil (Calan), hydrochlorothiazide (HydroDIURIL), and oral potassium chloride. He has not returned to your office since the initial diagnosis. During the past 12 months, he has reduced his weight from 280 lb to 198 lb using a rigorous exercise and diet program. Although he is proud of his lifestyle changes, he is complaining of fatigue, dizziness, heart palpitations, and muscle weakness.

    a. List two or three nursing diagnoses appropriate for Mr. S.

    b. What further assessment data should be obtained?

39. Ms. F, a 49-year-old television producer, works 70 hours per week and has recently been diagnosed with hypertension. Ms. F reports smoking one pack per day for the past 15 years. She is concerned about the new medication prescribed for her, spironolactone (Aldactone). She appears distressed yet in a hurry to return to work.

    a. What immediate goals are appropriate for Ms. F?

    b. What patient teaching is appropriate for Ms. F? Include teaching methods.

CHAPTER 44

DRUGS FOR FLUID, ELECTROLYTE, AND ACID-BASE DISORDERS

OBJECTIVES

To view the objectives, please refer to the textbook, student CD-ROM, and the Companion Website at *www.prenhall.com/adams*.

FILL IN THE BLANK

From the textbook, find the correct word(s) to complete the statements(s).

1. _____ are used to replace fluids that have been lost and to promote urine output.

2. When the body's pH drops below _____, acidosis occurs and symptoms of CNS depression are observed.

3. The normal pH of most body fluids is approximately _____.

4. Increasing the renal excretion of bicarbonate ion will increase the _____ of the blood.

5. _____ IV fluids cause water to move from the interstitial fluid to the plasma.

6. _____ IV fluids cause water to move from the plasma to the interstitial fluid.

7. _____ IV fluids produce no net fluid shift.

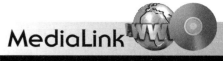

MediaLink

www.prenhall.com/adams

CD-ROM
Animations:
  Fluid Balance
  Acids
Audio Glossary
NCLEX Review

Companion Website
NCLEX Review
Dosage Calculations
Case Study
Care Plans
Expanded Key Concepts

MATCHING

For questions 8 through 12, match the drug in column I with its classification in column II.

Column I	Column II
8. _____ Dextran 70 (Macrodex)	a. Colloid
9. _____ 5% dextrose in water (D_5W)	b. Crystalloid
10. _____ Plasmalyte	
11. _____ Hetastarch (Hespan)	
12. _____ Lactated Ringer's	

MULTIPLE CHOICE

13. The nurse may begin to recognize symptoms of alkalosis at a pH above which of the following?

    a. 6.5

    b. 7.0

    c. 7.35

    d. 7.45

14. When acidosis is suspected, the healthcase provider should first assess for abnormalities in which body system?

    a. GI

    b. CNS

    c. Renal

    d. Cardiovascular

15. The nurse would expect to administer which of the following to a patient with alkalosis?

    a. Sodium bicarbonate

    b. Sodium chloride combined with potassium chloride

    c. Lithium carbonate

    d. Aluminum hydroxide

16. Which is the drug of choice for correcting acidosis?

    a. Sodium bicarbonate

    b. Sodium chloride

    c. Ammonium chloride

    d. Potassium chloride

17. Which is the drug of choice for treating or preventing hypokalemia?

    a. Sodium bicarbonate

    b. Sodium chloride

    c. Ammonium chloride

    d. Potassium chloride

18. The nurse should monitor for the most common side effect of oral potassium chloride. Which of the following is the most common?

    a. Drowsiness

    b. Nausea and vomiting

    c. Hypoglycemia

    d. Muscle weakness and fatigue

19. In severe cases, serum potassium levels may be quickly lowered by administration of which of the following?

    a. Glucose and insulin

    b. Furosemide (Lasix)

    c. Acetazolamide (Diamox)

    d. Sodium bicarbonate

20. Colloids cause water molecules to move from the tissues into the blood vessels through their ability to increase which of the following?

    a. Potassium levels

    b. Sodium levels

    c. Sodium excretion

    d. Osmotic pressure

21. Patients who need sodium replacement may be prescribed an IV solution containing which of the following?

    a. Large proteins

    b. Glucose

    c. Electrolytes

    d. Dextran

22. Which of the following patients may suffer from acidosis?

    a. 70-year-old with kidney failure

    b. 34-year-old who has ingested excess sodium bicarbonate

    c. 15-year-old with hyperventilation due to anxiety

    d. 57-year-old taking diuretics

23. Which of the following situations may lead to alkalosis?

    a. Hypoventilation or shallow breathing

    b. Severe vomiting

    c. Severe diarrhea

    d. Diabetes mellitus

24. The nurse correctly identifies hyponatremia when reviewing which of the following lab values?

    a. Sodium 133 mEq/L

    b. Sodium 148 mEq/L

    c. Potassium 3.5 mEq/L

    d. Potassium 5.5 mEq/L

25. The nurse should teach patients taking potassium supplements to take the drug according to which method?

    a. With no other medications

    b. An hour before or 2 hours after a meal

    c. With a meal

    d. In the morning, upon awakening

MAKING CONNECTIONS

26. Naldecon Senior DX is a combination drug consisting of dextromethorphan 10 mg and guaifenesin 200 mg. Naldecon is most likely prescribed for which of the following?

    a. Cold and flu symptoms

    b. Mild to moderate pain

    c. Asthma

    d. Hypertension

27. Alkylating agents such as cyclophosphamide (Cytoxan) are primarily used to treat which of the following?

    a. Immune disorders

    b. Severe inflammation

    c. Cancer

    d. HIV/AIDS

28. Which of the following is least likely to be caused by use of diuretics in the elderly patient?

    a. Incontinence

    b. Social isolation

    c. Depression

    d. Improved mental acuity

29. The nurse encourages intake of cranberry juice for a patient with frequent urinary tract infections because cranberries may do which of the following?

    a. Increase the urine acidity

    b. Decrease the urine acidity

    c. Increase hematocrit levels

    d. Decrease hematocrit levels

30. Which of the following is considered to be an intermediate-acting thiazide diuretic?

    a. Furosemide (Lasix)

    b. Metolazone (Zaroxolyn)

    c. Chlorothiazide (Diuril)

    d. Spironolactone (Aldactone)

CALCULATIONS

31. The physician ordered crystalloid solution 1000 cc 0.9% NaCl to infuse per pump over 8 hours. The nurse will set the pump at what rate?

32. The physician ordered ammonium chloride 8 g/d in divided doses q6h. The pharmacy sends 500 mg tablets. How many tablets will the nurse administer at each dose?

CASE STUDY APPLICATIONS

33. Ms. S decided to lose weight and chose a plan that eliminated almost all dietary carbohydrates. She has been taking hydrochlorothiazide and aspirin for her arthritis and potassium chloride. After 2 weeks, she can no longer endure the stomach pain, nausea, and cramping. Her husband reports that his wife has shown considerable fatigue and sleepiness.

    a. Analyze the assessment data to develop a nursing plan of care for Ms. S.

    b. What patient teaching is appropriate for Ms. S?

34. Mr. W, a 60-year-old utility worker, was admitted to the ER with symptoms of hyponatremia following an 8-hour workday. The environmental temperature averaged 75 degrees.

    a. What additional assessment data are important for the nurse to gather?

    b. What nursing interventions would be appropriate to assist Mr. W in avoiding hyponatremia in the future?

CHAPTER 45

DRUGS FOR MUSCLE SPASMS AND SPASTICITY

OBJECTIVES

To view the objectives, please refer to the textbook, student CD-ROM, and the Companion Website at *www.prenhall.com/adams*.

FILL IN THE BLANK

From the textbook, find the correct word(s) to complete the statement(s).

1. Disorders associated with _____ are some of the most difficult conditions to treat because of the mechanisms underlying them.

2. Movement disorders span the _____,

   _____, _____, and _____

   body systems.

3. Involuntary contractions of a muscle or group of muscles are called _____.

4. Pharmacotherapy used for muscle spasm usually includes _____, _____, and

   _____ drugs.

5. A muscle condition that results from damage to the CNS is _____.

6. A chronic neurologic disorder in which involuntary muscle contraction forces body parts into abnormal

   postures is _____.

7. Prolonged muscle spasms are referred to as _____.

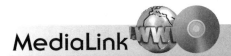

MediaLink

www.prenhall.com/adams

CD-ROM
Animation:
   Mechanism in Action: Cyclobenzaprine
      (Cycloflex, Flexeril)
Audio Glossary
NCLEX Review

Companion Website
NCLEX Review
Dosage Calculations
Case Study
Care Plans
Expanded Key Concepts

MATCHING

For questions 8 through 15, match the drug in column I with the letter for the drug classification in column II.

Column I	Column II
8. _____ Cyclobenzaprine (Flexeril)	a. Centrally acting antispasmodic
9. _____ Dantrolene (Dantrium)	b. Skeletal muscle relaxer
10. _____ Quinine sulfate (Quinamm)	
11. _____ Diazepam (Valium)	
12. _____ Chlorzoxazone (Parafon Forte)	
13. _____ Botulinum toxin A (Botox)	
14. _____ Carisoprodol (Soma)	
15. _____ Methocarbamol (Robaxin)	

MULTIPLE CHOICE

16. Causes of muscle spasms include all except which one?

    a. Overmedication with antipsychotic drugs

    b. Overdose of calcium

    c. Hypocalcemia

    d. Epilepsy

17. Nonpharmacologic measures that may be used to treat muscle spasms include all except which one?

    a. Encouraging use of the affected muscle

    b. Thermotherapy

    c. Hydrotherapy

    d. Ultrasound

18. Which of the following statements about cyclobenzaprine (Flexeril) is false?

    a. Its mechanism of action is similar to tricyclic antidepressants.

    b. It is effective in cerebral palsy.

    c. It is meant for short-term use.

    d. It is not recommended for use in children.

19. All of the following drugs are effective in the treatment of spasticity except which one?

    a. Baclofen

    b. Diazepam

    c. Dantrolene

    d. Cyclobenzaprine

20. How does botulinum toxin (Botox, Myobloc) produce its effects?

    a. It blocks the release of norepinephrine from nerve tissue.

b. It blocks the release of acetylcholine from cholinergic nerve terminals.

c. It increases the release of acetylcholine from cholinergic nerve terminals.

d. It increases the rate at which GABA is broken down in the body.

21. When teaching a patient receiving a centrally acting antispasmodic drug, which statement is incorrect?

    a. "You should avoid hazardous activities such as driving if the drug makes you drowsy."

    b. "You should avoid alcohol and antihistamines."

    c. "If you have severe side effects, stop taking the drug at once."

    d. "You should not take this drug if you have liver disease."

22. All of the following statements regarding dantrolene (Dantrium) are correct except which one?

    a. Its use is contraindicated in patients with malignant hyperthermia.

    b. It is useful in spasms of head and neck muscles.

    c. It is useful in cases of spinal cord injury or CVA.

    d. It does not affect cardiac or smooth muscle.

23. Which of the following statements best describes the etiology of tetany?

    a. Blood calcium levels are too low, leading to cell membranes being extremely excitable.

    b. Blood calcium levels are too high, leading to cell membranes being extremely excitable.

    c. Blood potassium levels are too low, leading to cell membranes being extremely excitable.

    d. Blood calcium levels are too low, leading to cell membranes being extremely lethargic.

24. Which of these drugs is produced by bacteria and is responsible for food poisoning in high quantities?

    a. Dantrolene

    b. Botulinum toxin

    c. Quinine sulfate

    d. Diazepam

25. Which of the following drug classes increases the risk of unfavorable reactions to antispasmodics?

    a. MAO inhibitors

    b. Pain medications

    c. Antibiotics

    d. Anticonvulsants

26. Patients who abruptly discontinue baclofen (Lioresal) may experience which of the following?

    a. Palpitations, chest pain, dyspnea

    b. Urinary retention

    c. Hallucinations, paranoia, and seizures

    d. Dry mouth and photosensitivity

27. Your patient reports to you that in addition to the drug therapy provided by his nurse, he is using cayenne (*Capsicum annum*) for his muscle spasms. Which precaution should this patient take?

    a. Wear sun block lotion and long sleeves.

    b. Never apply to broken skin.

    c. Do not use this substance if you use any alcohol.

    d. If you notice any urinary hesitancy, discontinue use at once.

MAKING CONNECTIONS

28. What is the neurotransmitter for skeletal muscle contraction?

    a. Acetylcholine

    b. Serotonin

    c. Norepinephrine

    d. Epinephrine

29. Which normal physiological action other than muscle contraction depends on calcium?

    a. Relaxation of blood vessels

    b. Termination of neurotransmitter action

    c. Transmission of a pain impulse

    d. Blood coagulation

30. Vitamin D can be synthesized from which of the following chemicals?

    a. Triglycerides

    b. Steroids

    c. Protein

    d. Bile

31. Which of the following vitamins is also known as cyanocobalamin?

    a. A

    b. B_{12}

    c. C

    d. K

32. Which of the following statements about NSAIDs is false?

    a. They are used to decrease inflammation after injuries.

    b. They include aspirin, ibuprofen, naproxen, and acetaminophen.

    c. One of their main side effects is GI upset.

    d. They are used to treat fever.

CALCULATIONS

33. The patient has an order for dantrolene (Dantrium) 75 mg bid. On hand are tablets labeled "dantrolene 25 mg." How many tablets should the nurse give for each dose? How many mg will the nurse give per day?

34. The patient has an order for cyclobenzaprine (Flexeril) 20 mg tid. On hand are tablets labeled "cyclobenzaprine 10 mg." How many tablets should the nurse give for each dose? Is this a safe dose?

CASE STUDY APPLICATIONS

35. Ms. H has been experiencing lower back pain for 2 months due to muscle spasms. So far, no other disorders have been identified that could explain this pain. Her doctor has prescribed cyclobenzaprine (Flexeril).

   a. Describe other nondrug therapy that might help in this case.

   b. When teaching Ms. H about adverse reactions to cyclobenzaprine, what information should be included?

   c. How will the nurse determine whether this drug is effective?

   d. Prior to discharge, your goal is to have the patient state ways to prevent recurrence of her symptoms. What preventive teaching should be done for this patient?

36. Your patient, Ms. B, has a career as a model and fashion designer. She expresses concern over the "crow's feet and frown lines" she's beginning to develop. She asks for information on the new Botox injections she has heard about. She expresses concern over the fact that she's heard they use a "poison" to remove facial wrinkles but says "it would be great to look 16 again!" Your nursing diagnosis is knowledge deficit related to use of cosmetic procedures, and teaching is a planned intervention.

   a. What misinformation do you need to correct when talking with this patient?

   b. What side effects does Ms. B need to be aware of before having the Botox injections?

37. Mr. P is a 21-year-old patient with cerebral palsy who is cared for at home by his parents. His mother expresses concern over his spasticity and wants "better drugs" to control it. He is currently using Lioresal.

   a. What assessments should be done on Mr. P?

   b. What nondrug therapy might be useful for Mr. P?

   c. What patient/family teaching should be done regarding Mr. P's use of antispasmodic drugs at home?

   d. What patient/family teaching should be done regarding nondrug and safety interventions for Mr. P?

CHAPTER 46

DRUGS FOR BONE AND JOINT DISORDERS

OBJECTIVES

To view the objectives, please refer to the textbook, student CD-ROM, and the Companion Website at *www.prenhall.com/adams*.

FILL IN THE BLANK

From the textbook, find the correct word(s) to complete the statement(s).

1. One of the most important minerals in the body responsible for
   bone formation is _____.

2. Calcium levels in the bloodstream are controlled by two
   endocrine glands, the _____ glands and the _____ gland.

3. Calcium disorders are often related to _____ disorders.

4. Osteomalacia, referred to as _____ in children, is a disorder characterized by softening of bones
   without alteration of basic bone structure.

5. Two important disorders characterized by weak and fragile bones are _____ and _____,

6. The hormone responsible for bone resorption is _____; the hormone responsible for bone
   deposition is _____.

7. Cholecalciferol is converted to an intermediate vitamin form called _____; this intermediate form
   is transported to the kidneys where enzymes transform it into _____ an active form of vitamin D.

8. The two major forms of calcium used in pharmacotherapy are _____ and _____.

---

9. _____ is a class of drugs that provides the same protection against uterine or breast cancer as progesterone in estrogen replacement therapy (ERT).

10. A class of drugs called _____ is chemically similar to natural bisphosphates found in body tissues.

11. Two drug therapies for Paget's disease are _____ and _____.

12. _____ treat rheumatoid arthritis by suppressing autoimmunity.

13. Drugs preventing the accumulation of uric acid in the bloodstream or joint cavities are

    called _____.

MATCHING

For questions 14 through 20, match the drug in column I with its classification in column II.

Column I	Column II
14. _____ Calcitriol (Calcijex, Rocaltrol)	a. Calcium supplement
15. _____ Calcium carbonate (BioCal)	b. Vitamin D therapy
16. _____ Allopurinol (Lopurin, Zyloprim)	c. Inhibitor of bone resorption
17. _____ Etidronate disodium (Didronel)	d. Disease-modifying drug
18. _____ Aurothioglucose (Gold thioglucose, Solganal)	e. Uric acid inhibitor
19. _____ Colchicine	
20. _____ Alendronate (Fosamax)	

For questions 21 through 25 match the indication in column I with its drug in column II.

Column I	Column II
21. _____ Osteomalacia, rickets, and hypocalcemia	a. Alendronate sodium (Fosamax)
22. _____ Osteoporosis, Paget's disease	b. Probenecid (Benemid)
23. _____ Gouty arthritis	c. Ergocalciferol (Deltalin, Calciferol)
24. _____ Rheumatoid arthritis	d. Hydroxychloroquine sulfate (Plaquenil Sulfate)
25. _____ Osteoarthritis	e. Sodium hyaluronate (Hyalgan)

MULTIPLE CHOICE

26. Which of the following statements regarding calcium in the body is false?

    a. When concentrations are too high, sodium permeability decreases across cell membranes.

    b. When concentrations are too low, cell membranes become hyperexcitable.

    c. Calcium must be present for the body to form vitamin D.

    d. Calcium is important for body processes such as blood coagulation and muscle contraction.

27. Diseases and conditions of calcium and vitamin D metabolism include all except which one?

    a. Osteomalacia

    b. Rheumatoid arthritis

    c. Osteoporosis

    d. Paget's disease

28. Possible etiologies of hypocalcemia include all except which one?

    a. Hyposecretion of parathyroid hormone

    b. Digestive-related malabsorption disorders

    c. Lack of adequate intake of calcium-containing foods

    d. Paget's disease

29. You are helping your elderly patient who has osteoporosis mark her menu. Which of the following choices would be *least* useful in helping her maintain adequate calcium intake?

    a. Carton of milk for breakfast

    b. Salmon croquette for dinner

    c. Turnip greens for dinner

    d. Baked potato for lunch

30. Calcium gluconate is contraindicated in patients with all of the following conditions except which one?

    a. Osteomalacia

    b. Digitalis toxicity

    c. Kidney stones

    d. Cardiac dysrhythmia

31. Patient teaching regarding vitamin D therapy includes all except which one?

    a. Take exactly as directed; it can become toxic if taken in excess quantities.

    b. Avoid alcohol and other hepatotoxic drugs.

    c. Avoid sunlight exposure due to susceptibility to sunburn.

    d. Do not start a low-fat diet unless first discussed with nurse.

32. All of the following are risk for factors for osteoporosis except which one?

    a. Anorexia nervosa

    b. Use of estrogen replacement therapy

    c. High alcohol or caffeine consumption

    d. Advancing age in women

33. Which statement regarding calcitonin is false?

    a. Obtained from salmon

    b. Currently available only in oral form

   c. Increases bone density and reduces the incidence of vertebral fractures

   d. Indicated for Paget's disease and hypercalcemia

34. Selective estrogen receptor modulators (SERMs) are contraindicated in patients with all of the following conditions except which one?

   a. Thromboembolism

   b. Pregnancy or lactation

   c. Hormone replacement

   d. Postmenopause

35. Which of the following is *not* a symptom of osteomalacia and/or rickets?

   a. Hypocalcemia

   b. Convulsions

   c. Muscle weakness

   d. Bowlegs and a pigeon breast

36. After analgesic and anti-inflammatory drugs have been tried, which of the following therapies may be used to alter the course of rheumatoid arthritis progression?

   a. Bisphosphonates

   b. Calcitonin therapy

   c. Disease-modifying drugs

   d. Uric acid inhibitors

37. Which of the following gout medications is used for an acute attack and may cause gastric upset?

   a. Colchicine

   b. Allopurinol (Lopurin)

   c. Penicillamine (Cuprimine, Depen)

   d. Sulfasalazine (Azulfidine)

38. Sodium hyaluronate (Hyalgan) is a new therapy for patients with moderate osteoarthritis. Which statement about this drug is false?

   a. It is injected directly into the knee joint.

   b. It coats the articulating cartilage surface.

   c. Patients should avoid strenuous activity for 48 hours after it is administered.

   d. It is used prior to treatments with COX-2 inhibitors and NSAIDs.

39. Which of the following patients is least likely to present with gout?

   a. Pacific Islander

   b. Male

   c. Female

   d. Patient using a thiazide diuretic

MAKING CONNECTIONS

40. Methotrexate can be used to treat rheumatoid arthritis. What other condition is it used for?

    a. Cancer

    b. Pernicious anemia

    c. Cardiac dysrhythmia

    d. Renal failure

41. Promethazine (Phenergan) is a phenothiazine that is used to treat which of the following?

    a. Dysrhythmia

    b. Hypertension

    c. Inflammation

    d. Motion sickness

42. In addition to treating rheumatoid arthritis, hydroxychloroquine (Plaquenil) is also used for which of the following?

    a. Cancer

    b. Pernicious anemia

    c. Malaria

    d. Renal failure

43. Isoniazid can affect serum calcium by causing hypercalcemia. A patient receiving this drug is being treated for which disease?

    a. Peptic ulcers

    b. Tuberculosis infection

    c. Viral infection

    d. Inflammation

44. Diazepam (Valium) is used as an antianxiety agent in many hospitalized patients. What other condition is it used for?

    a. Muscle spasms

    b. Osteomyelitis

    c. Parkinson's disease

    d. Immune disorders

CALCULATIONS

45. The nurse is giving colchicine 0.5 mg tablets for an acute attack of gout. The dose is to be repeated every hour until the patient develops GI symptoms or the pain is relieved. The maximum dose is 4 mg. How many doses can the nurse give before the maximum dose is reached?

46. Hydroxychloroquine sulfate (Plaquenil) 400 mg daily is ordered for a patient with rheumatoid arthritis. Available are 200 mg tablets. How many tablets should be given?

CASE STUDY APPLICATIONS

47. Your patient is a 74-year-old male who has primary gout and has just started taking allopurinol (Lopurin), 100 mg daily. He is reporting symptoms of gastric upset and intermittent episodes of extreme pain in the joints.

    a. What education should the nurse provide regarding these symptoms and their treatment?

    b. What education should the nurse provide regarding possible adverse effects?

    c. What laboratory tests should the nurse monitor to determine the longer term effects of allopurinol?

48. Ms. S is a 28-year-old type I diabetic with renal failure on hemodialysis. You bring her AM medications which include Rocaltrol and calcium tablets.

    a. She asks you why she is receiving vitamin D and calcium since she does not have a bone disease and is too young for osteoporosis. How do you explain this to her?

    b. What patient teaching regarding vitamin D therapy would you give Ms. S?

    c. What information regarding calcium supplements should you give her?

49. Mrs. R is 78 years old and has been admitted to the hospital with a vertebral compression fracture. Now that her pain has been controlled, she is asking you questions about prevention of further problems of this nature.

    a. Mrs. R wants to know what causes the bones to come brittle in elderly people. What explanation will you give her?

    b. What drug therapy is likely to be prescribed to treat Mrs. R's osteoporosis?

    c. What education will Mrs. R need regarding the use of her prescriptions for Fosamax and Evista?

CHAPTER 47

DRUGS FOR SKIN DISORDERS

OBJECTIVES

To view the objectives, please refer to the textbook, student CD-ROM, and the Companion Website at *www.prenhall.com/adams*.

FILL IN THE BLANK

From the textbook, find the correct word(s) to complete the statement(s).

1. Drugs used to promote the shedding of old skin are called

   _____ agents.

2. Mites cause a skin disorder called _____.

3. Vitamin A–like compounds providing resistance to bacterial infection by reducing oil production

   and the occurrence of clogged pores are called _____.

4. Drugs used to soothe and soften the skin, as in the case of psoriasis,

   are called _____.

5. Itching associated with dry, scaly skin is called _____.

6. Other than keratolytic agents, two classes of drugs offer some protection against acne,

   including _____ and _____.

7. A skin disorder with symptoms resembling an allergic reaction is called atopic

   dermatitis or _____.

8. Small inflammatory bumps without pus are called _____.

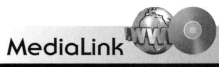

MediaLink

www.prenhall.com/adams

CD-ROM
Audio Glossary
NCLEX Review

Companion Website
NCLEX Review
Dosage Calculations
Case Study
Care Plans
Expanded Key Concepts

MATCHING

For questions 9 through 15, match the drug in column I with its classification in column II.

Column I	**Column II**
9. _____ Benzoyl peroxide (BenzaClin)	a. Scabicide/pediculicide
10. _____ Fluticasone (Flonase)	b. Sunburn/minor irritation agent
11. _____ Etretinate (Tegison)	c. Acne and acne-related agent
12. _____ Azelaic acid (Azelex)	d. Topical glucocorticoid
13. _____ Lindane (Kwell)	e. Psoriatic agent
14. _____ Benzocaine (Solarcaine)	
15. _____ Sulfacetamide sodium (AK-Sulf)	

For questions 16 through 20, match the symptom in column I with its description in column II.

Column I	**Column II**
16. _____ Erythema	a. Blackheads
17. _____ Pruritus	b. Whiteheads
18. _____ Sunburn	c. Intense itching
19. _____ Open comedones	d. Redness
20. _____ Closed comedones	e. "First-degree" injury

MULTIPLE CHOICE

21. Drugs to treat oily skin would most likely be used for which of the following disorders?

    a. Atopic dermatitis

    b. Contact dermatitis

    c. Seborrheic dermatitis

    d. Stasis dermatitis

22. Which of the following medications is also used for the treatment of wrinkles?

    a. Benzoyl peroxide (BenzaClin)

    b. Tretinoin (Retin-A)

    c. Calcipotriene (Dovonex)

    d. Hydroxyurea (Hydrea)

23. Which of the following medications is administered topically for psoriasis?

    a. Calcipotriene (Dovonex)

    b. Acitretin (Soriatane)

    c. Etretinate (Tegison)

    d. Methotrexate (Amethopterin, Folex, Rheumatrex)

24. Which of the following medications would *not* be useful for minor insect bites?

    a. Benzocaine (Solarcaine)

    b. Dibucaine (Nupercainal)

    c. Tetracaine (Pontocaine)

    d. Isotretinoin (Accutane)

25. Which of the following treatments would *not* be used to promote the shedding of old skin?

    a. Resorcinol

    b. Salicylic acid

    c. Sulfur

    d. Benzoyl peroxide

26. Which of the following statements about benzocaine is true?

    a. When applied to the ear, mouth, or throat, it produces minor irritation.

    b. It is more appropriate for sunburn than for pruritus or insect bites.

    c. Drug sensitivity is rare.

    d. It should not be applied to an open wound.

27. Which of the following is an over-the-counter medication for acne?

    a. Adapalene (Differin)

    b. Azelaic acid (Azelex)

    c. Benzoyl peroxide (BenzaClin)

    d. Sulfacetamide (Klaron)

28. Exposure to perfume, cosmetics, detergents, or latex is associated with which of the following disorders?

    a. Atopic dermatitis

    b. Contact dermatitis

    c. Seborrheic dermatitis

    d. Stasis dermatitis

29. Topical glucocorticoids are a common treatment for all of the following except which one?

    a. Psoriasis

    b. Rosacea

    c. Pruritus

    d. Dermatitis

30. Which of the following is contraindicated in conjunction with phototherapy for the treatment of psoriasis?

    a. Tar and anthralin

    b. Keratolytic pastes

    c. Psoralens

    d. Cyclosporine

31. Lindane (Kwell) is contraindicated in all of the following patients except which one?

    a. Children ages 2–10

    b. Children less than 2 years old

    c. Children with seizures

    d. Children who have abrasions, rash, or dermatitis

32. Use of Accutane is contraindicated in patients with all of these conditions except which one?

    a. Rosacea

    b. Severe depression and suicidal tendencies

    c. Seizures treated with carbamazepine

    d. Diabetes treated with oral agents

33. Which vitamin is synthesized by the skin?

    a. Vitamin A

    b. Vitamin D

    c. Vitamin E

    d. Vitamin K

MAKING CONNECTIONS

34. Methotrexate may be used to treat psoriasis. Which other condition is it used for?

    a. Gout and rheumatoid arthritis

    b. Rheumatoid arthritis and certain cancers

    c. Systemic fungal infections and certain cancers

    d. Urinary tract infections and peptic ulcers

35. Topical metronidazole (Flagyl) is used to treat rosacea. What condition is it used for when given PO or IV?

    a. Crohn's disease

    b. To decrease lipid levels in the blood

    c. Anti-infective therapy

    d. Dysrhythmia

36. What drug is used as a local anesthetic and an antidysrhythmic?

    a. Warfarin (Coumadin)

    b. Propranolol (Inderal)

    c. Infliximab (Remicade)

    d. Lidocaine (Xylocaine)

37. Which is among the first-line drugs used for allergic rhinitis?

    a. NSAIDs

    b. Sympathomimetics

    c. Glucocorticoids

    d. Cytokines

CASE STUDY APPLICATIONS

38. Ms. G is a 9-year-old brought to the pediatrician by her mother for an immunization. As you give the injection you notice that the child has nits clinging to her hair. A quick assessment tells you that the child appears to be clean and well cared for. When you point out the problem to her mother, she confesses that she has used an OTC treatment for the lice, which her daughter got at a friend's sleepover. She is obviously uncomfortable and blurts out, "We're not like that—we are clean people." A prescription for Kwell is given to the mother.

    a. What teaching must you do regarding the use of lindane?

    b. Whom must the mother notify of her daughter's pediculosis?

    c. What information can you give mother and daughter to prevent this problem from recurring?

39. You are working at a walk-in clinic in Florida. A 20-year-old college student visiting from Minnesota on spring break presents with complaints of severe sunburn.

    a. What other assessments would you need?

    b. What interventions might help the pain and other symptoms of sunburn?

    c. Promotion of wellness is one goal in your care plan. What information should be given to the young man regarding prevention and sequelae of sunburn?

40. Zack, a 17-year-old, stops by the school nurse's office to "hang out." After some preliminary conversation he confides to you that he is worried about his complexion, and that nothing he has tried has cleared up his severe acne. He is afraid he will be "scarred for life" and asks if there are any other medications to help him. He also wants to know why he has such a bad case of acne, and his friend has hardly any.

    a. What can you tell Zack about the causes of acne?

    b. What assessments must be made prior to starting Accutane?

    c. What other information should be assessed regarding Zack's lifestyle and hygiene habits?

CHAPTER 48

DRUGS FOR EYE AND EAR DISORDERS

OBJECTIVES

To view the objectives, please refer to the textbook, student CD-ROM, and the Companion Website at *www.prenhall.com/adams*.

FILL IN THE BLANK

From the textbook, find the correct word(s) to complete the statement(s).

1. In patients who have glaucoma, increased intraocular pressure

   is most often caused by a _____ in the

   _____ of aqueous humor.

2. A type of slower developing glaucoma where the iris does not cover the trabecular meshwork

   is referred to as _____.

3. Drugs that cause the pupils to constrict are called _____.

4. Drugs that cause the pupils to dilate are referred to as _____.

5. Drugs that cause relaxation of ciliary muscles are called _____.

6. Swimmer's ear is sometimes referred to as _____.

7. Inflammation of the middle ear is called _____.

8. Inflammation of the mastoid sinus is called _____.

9. Another word for earwax is _____.

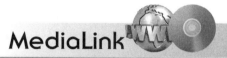

MediaLink

www.prenhall.com/adams

CD-ROM
Animation:
   Mechanism in Action: Pilocarpine
Audio Glossary
NCLEX Review

Companion Website
NCLEX Review
Dosage Calculations
Case Study
Care Plans
Expanded Key Concepts

MATCHING

For questions 10 through 15, match the drug in column I with its action in column II.

Column I	Column II
10. _____ Pilocarpine HCl (Adsorbocarpine)	a. Increase the outflow of aqueous humor
11. _____ Timolol (Timoptic)	b. Decrease the formation of aqueous humor
12. _____ Acetazolamide (Diamox)	
13. _____ Mannitol (Osmitrol)	
14. _____ Epinephrine borate (Epinal)	
15. _____ Latanoprost (Xalatan)	

For questions 16 through 23, match the antiglaucoma drug in column I with its classification in column II.

Column I	Column II
16. _____ Pilocarpine (Adsorbocarpine)	a. Miotic, direct-acting cholinergic agonist
17. _____ Dorzolamide HCl (Trusopt)	b. Miotic, cholinesterase inhibitor
18. _____ Isosorbide (Ismotic)	c. Sympathomimetic
19. _____ Epinephrine borate (Epinal)	d. Prostaglandin or prostamide
20. _____ Demecarium bromide (Humorsol)	e. Beta-blocker
21. _____ Travaprost (Travatan)	f. Alpha$_2$-adrenergic agonist, direct acting
22. _____ Betaxolol (Betoptic)	g. Carbonic anhydrase inhibitor
23. _____ Apraclonidine (Iopidine)	h. Osmotic diuretic

MULTIPLE CHOICE

24. Which of the following types of medications may contribute to the development of glaucoma?

   a. Beta-blockers

   b. Glucocorticoids

   c. Antibiotics

   d. Calcium channel blockers

25. Which of the following best describes closed-angle glaucoma?

   a. Is referred to as chronic, simple glaucoma

   b. Develops when the iris is pushed over the area where the aqueous fluid normally drains

   c. Develops more slowly than open-angle glaucoma

   d. Is best treated by drugs that decrease the formation of aqueous humor

26. Which of the following classes of drugs for eye procedures should *not* be used for patients with glaucoma?

   a. Mydriatic (sympathomimetic) drugs

   b. Cycloplegic (anticholinergic) drugs

    c. Osmotic diuretics

    d. Carbonic anhydrase inhibitors

27. When used for glaucoma, one drawback of prostaglandins is that they do which of the following?

    a. Change pigmentation of the eye

    b. Reduce blood pressure

    c. Increase urine output

    d. Block sympathetic impulses

28. Which of the following medications is converted to epinephrine in the eye?

    a. Unoprostone isopropyl (Rescula)

    b. Physostigmine sulfate (Eserine sulfate)

    c. Dipivefrin hydrochloride (Propine)

    d. Echothiophate iodide (Phospholine iodide)

29. Which class of drugs used for eye examinations has the potential to produce unfavorable CNS effects?

    a. Osmotic diuretics

    b. Sympathomimetic drugs

    c. Anticholinergic drugs

    d. Cholinergic agonists

30. Major risk factors associated with glaucoma include all except which one?

    a. Hypertension

    b. Migraine headaches

    c. Ethnic origin

    d. Epilepsy

31. Which of the following statements regarding closed-angle (acute) glaucoma is false?

    a. It is usually unilateral.

    b. The iris is pushed over the area where the fluid normally drains.

    c. It is frequently seen in persons of Caucasian race.

    d. It constitutes an emergency situation.

32. Which of the following statements regarding beta-blocking agents is false?

    a. They are contraindicated in persons who are allergic to sulfa.

    b. They are the most frequently used antiglaucoma drug.

    c. The mechanism by which they work is not fully understood.

    d. They may produce systemic side effects such as bronchoconstriction, bradycardia, and hypotension.

33. In which patient would the use of Diamox, a carbonic anhydrase inhibitor, be contraindicated?

    a. A patient with asthma-producing bronchospasms

    b. A patient with an allergy to sulfonamides

    c. A patient with open-angle glaucoma

    d. A patient with a history of third-degree AV block

34. You are teaching an elderly patient to instill her own eye drops. How will you explain the procedure?

    a. Tilt the head back and toward the side of the affected eye.

    b. Tilt the head back and toward the side of the unaffected eye.

    c. Instill the drops to the center of the cornea, blink, and wipe the eye.

    d. Lift the upper lid by the lashes, and drop the medication into the sac.

35. When teaching a family member to instill eye drops for an elderly patient, you will include all except which one?

    a. Apply gentle pressure for 30 seconds to the inner canthus after instilling.

    b. Wait 5 minutes before instilling another type of drops.

    c. There is no need to remove the patient's contact lenses.

    d. Eye medication should be refrigerated.

36. What is the basic course of treatment for ear infection?

    a. Antibiotics

    b. Corticosteroids

    c. Earwax removal agents

    d. Irrigation with a bulb syringe

37. Which of the following regarding chloramphenicol (Chloromycetin Otic) ear drops is false?

    a. It is used primarily in cases of ruptured eardrum.

    b. It is indicated if the patient has hypersensitivity to the drug.

    c. It is the most commonly used topical antibiotic.

    d. Side effects include burning, redness, rash, and swelling.

38. When instilling ear drops, all of the following are correct except which one?

    a. Run warm water over the bottle to warm the drops.

    b. In an adult patient, the pinna should be held up and back.

    c. The patient should lie on the side opposite the affected ear for 5 minutes after instillation.

    d. The area should not be massaged to prevent systemic drug effects.

MAKING CONNECTIONS

39. Cholinergic agonists exert an effect in the body through which type of receptor?

    a. Nicotinic

    b. Muscarinic

    c. Dopaminergic

    d. Serotonergic

40. Beta-blockers are examples of which class of antidysrhythmic drugs?

    a. Class I

    b. Class II

    c. Class III

    d. Class IV

41. What is one important respiratory effect of beta-blockers?

    a. Bronchospasm

    b. Bronchodilation

    c. Increased release of surfactant

    d. Hyperventilation

42. What is the most serious adverse effect of taking potassium-sparing diuretics and salt substitutes at the same time?

    a. Hyperkalemia

    b. Hypokalemia

    c. Edema

    d. Dehydration

43. In addition to glaucoma, the carbonic anhydrase inhibitor acetazolamide (Diamox) is also prescribed for which of the following?

    a. Seizures

    b. Coagulation disorders

    c. Psoriasis

    d. Malaria

CALCULATIONS

44. The patient has an order for acetazolamide (Diamox) 250 mg, PO tid. What is the total amount of Diamox the patient will receive in 24 hours?

45. The patient has acute glaucoma. Pilocarpine HCl (Isopto Carpine) has been ordered 1 drop every 5 minutes for 6 doses. Would the nurse question this order? Why or why not?

CASE STUDY APPLICATIONS

46. Mr. M was recently diagnosed with open-angle glaucoma. Intraocular pressure is currently being controlled with miotic medications, including latanoprost (Xalatan). Mr. M wants to know if there is a permanent cure and if continued treatment will be necessary.

    a. Your care plan includes interventions related to patient education. What patient teaching must you do for Mr. M regarding his disease?

    b. One of Mr. M's nursing diagnoses reads "Knowledge deficit related to therapeutic regimen as evidenced by patient's inability to tell indications and side effects of antiglaucoma medications". What specific information regarding the use of latanoprost (Xalatan) must you give Mr. M?

    c. List some general nursing interventions that would be important for a patient with glaucoma.

    d. How would the nurse evaluate the effectiveness of Mr. M's glaucoma medications?

47. Five-year-old Timmy B is brought to the pediatrician's office by his mother who states he has been crying, running a temperature of 102°F, and complaining of an earache. Your assessment reveals bulging, reddened eardrums, and bloody drainage in the left ear. The mother states that she has been using chewable baby aspirin for his fever, and that she has another child at home using "ear drops, and he hates those cold things going into his ears." A diagnosis of otitis media is made by the doctor, and an oral antibiotic is prescribed.

    a. What other assessments must you make regarding the use of antibiotics by this patient?

    b. Mrs. B obviously has a lack of knowledge about Timmy's medications and treatments. What interventions could you include in your care plan to address this patient problem?

48. Mrs. I has come to the clinic with complaints of mild hearing loss and a sensation of fullness with intermittent ringing of the ears. Upon assessment with the otoscope, you observe a dark mass in the ear canal.

    a. What other assessments should be made prior to treating this problem?

    b. How would the problem be treated?

ANSWER KEY

Chapter 1

1. herbal
2. John Abel
3. chemists, active agents
4. synthesize
5. improving
6. study, medicines
7. prevention
8. prevention, treatment
9. therapeutic, adverse
10. Over-the-counter
11. b   12. c   13. a   14. d   15. b   16. a
17. c   18. d   19. c   20. d   21. d   22. c
23. d   24. b   25. c   26. d   27. d   28. a
29. a. It is important to cover the following points in a teaching plan for a patient with mild constipation.
    1. Natural alternatives usually cost less then OTC drugs.
    2. Natural alternatives tend to produce fewer side effects.
    3. Mild constipation can also be treated with diet changes: Try using high-fiber products and increasing water consumption.
    4. If constipation persists, the patient needs to make an appointment for assessment with a nurse.

    b. A nursing history would include the patient's medical history including bowel health, nutritional history, and medication history. It is important to evaluate what OTC medications have been taken in the past and what prescription drugs are being taken. Remember to assess both current and past herbal and alternative therapies. Also assess social history which includes use of alcohol, tobacco, and street drugs.
30. a. A patient can have a drug reaction to OTC, generic, or trade name medications. The important nursing action is to assess what reaction the patient is having and how life threatening it is for her. Life-threatening reactions include heart and lungs. If the patient is having difficulty breathing or is having a blood pressure or heart abnormality, then she needs to seek emergency care. All drug reactions should be taken seriously. A nurse should be consulted for all drug reactions.

    b. It is important for Ms. B to know that all prescription drugs are thoroughly tested because of the Food, Drug and Cosmetic Act of 1938. The Food and Drug Administration (FDA) must approve a drug before it is sold in the United States. The FDA also oversees administration of herbal products and dietary supplements. The Federal Trade Commission ensures that the advertising of OTC medications and health food supplements is not fraudulent, deceptive, or unsubstantiated.

Chapter 2

1. therapeutic
2. pharmacologic
3. prototype
4. chemical, generic, trade
5. chemical
6. generic
7. combination drugs
8. bioavailability
9. diphenhydramine
10. expensive
11. b   12. a   13. d   14. c   15. a   16. b
17. d   18. a   19. b   20. a   21. a   22. d
23. c   24. c
25. a. Generic and trade products have identical doses; however, the ingredients in the generic product may be slightly different. In many states, the pharmacist is allowed to dispense generic equivalents unless the patient or nurse specifies that a trade product is required. In Florida, if a drug is on the negative drug formulary list, it must be dispensed in its trade form only. As a nurse, it is best to check the state requirements for dispensing of trade versus generic products.

    b. Tylenol is an analgesic nonnarcotic. It is not a controlled substance. In the United States, controlled substances are drugs whose use is restricted by the Controlled Substances Act of 1970.

Chapter 3

1. influenza, tuberculosis, cholera, HIV
2. Strategic National Stockpile (SNS)
3. Push packages
4. hooves
5. protective antibodies
6. atropine
7. 3 to 4 hours

8. a	9. c	10. b	11. b	12. a	13. c
14. b	15. a	16. b	17. d	18. c	19. e
20. e	21. b	22. d	23. c	24. a	25. d
26. b	27. b	28. b	29. c	30. c	31. d

32. a

33. a. Because Mrs. M has not been exposed to anthrax, antibiotic use is not recommended. The antibiotic is expensive, can cause significant side effects, and, most importantly, can promote the development of bacterial strains that are resistant to antibiotics.

    b. Anthrax vaccine is available. It takes 18 months to complete the six injections. At this point, the CDC recommends vaccination for only laboratory personnel who work with anthrax, military personnel in high-risk areas, and those who deal with animal products imported from areas where the disease is endemic.

34. a. Assessments include checking for history of eczema, atopic dermatitis, and other exfoliative skin conditions, or patients who have the disease at present; checking for an alteration in immunity (HIV, AIDS, leukemia, lymphoma, immunosuppressive drugs); pregnancy or breastfeeding; age of the patient; and previous allergic reaction to any component of the vaccine.

    b. Information included in a pamphlet should include:
       1. The vaccine provides high-level protection if given prior to exposure or up to 3 days later.
       2. Protection may last from 3 to 5 years.
       3. The vaccine is contraindicated in people with serious skin conditions, immunocompromised persons, pregnancy, lactation, children under the age of 1 year, and anyone allergic to its components *unless* there is a documented face-to-face contact with an infected person.
       4. This vaccine is known for serious side effects. Of every million people vaccinated, 250 could die from the vaccine.

33. a. Potassium iodide prevents damage to the thyroid gland *only* after radiation exposure. It *does not* protect any other body tissues. It will not prevent radiation sickness or other cancers that may develop as a result of the exposure.

    b. Potassium iodide will be absorbed by the thyroid gland and prevent the radioactive iodine from being absorbed by the gland. This lessens the gland's exposure to radiation and prevents the cancer. KI is effective even if taken 3 to 4 hours after exposure.

Chapter 4

1. enteral
2. topical
3. pharmacokinetic
4. Viscosity, solubility
5. oral
6. Sublingual
7. Suppositories, enemas
8. intravenous
9. intramuscular
10. intrathecal, epidural
11. transdermal
12. Transmucosal

13. a	14. b	15. b	16. a	17. c	18. b
19. c	20. a	21. b	22. b	23. b	24. c
25. a	26. a	27. b	28. b	29. c	30. a
31. b	32. a	33. c	34. b	35. d	36. d
37. c	38. d	39. a	40. b	41. b	42. b
43. c	44. d	45. b	46. d	47. c	

48. a. The nurse must take a detailed personal, family, and sexual health history when assisting the patient in a choice of contraception.

    b. Oral contraceptive agents are effective and convenient; however, missing a daily dose means risking pregnancy. Therefore, for an active lifestyle, this may not be the most desirable approach. On the other hand, an oral medication may be less bothersome than injections, patches, or vaginal inserts. Injections or implants may last a long time, but they may be initially painful or subject to infection. In addition, these approaches may be uncomfortable, as may vaginal inserts. Vaginal inserts might be used less routinely because they are sometimes messy, inconvenient, and less reliable. The nurse should help the patient weigh every disadvantage against the convenience of taking medication less frequently.

49. a. Because the patient is nauseous and has diarrhea, oral medications or suppositories would probably not be recommended unless the nausea and diarrhea were not severe enough to interfere with the drug therapy. Because the source of discomfort is the gastrointestinal tract, topical drugs would most likely do little good to relieve discomfort; and in elderly patients, the skin is usually sensitive. Alternatives might be drugs administered by the parenteral route, for example, in an intramuscular or subcutaneous injection.

    b. Effectiveness of the route of medication can be evaluated by collecting data about the resolution of presenting symptoms.

Chapter 5

1. absorption, distribution, metabolism, excretion
2. blood-brain, fetal-placental
3. Metabolism
4. first-pass effect
5. Absorption
6. bone marrow, teeth, eyes, adipose tissue
7. excretion
8. Toxic concentration
9. therapeutic range
10. loading
11. a   12. b   13. a   14. b   15. a   16. b
17. c   18. b   19. c   20. a   21. a   22. c
23. d   24. a
25. a. Because Mr. P is obese, the medications may be dissolved in the fat and accumulate there, and then slowly be released. Hypertension and diabetes can alter drug distribution as these disorders are associated with compromised renal function. When renal function is compromised, drug dosing must be reduced to account for changes in metabolic and excretion function.

    b. Mr. P's anxiety should be reduced. Half-life of the drug should be considered by the nurse. If the patient is experiencing side effects of the antianxiety drugs, then the nurse should consider renal and hepatic function as a potential problem, increasing the plasma half-life.

    c. The primary site of excretion for all medications is the kidney. The nurse should be checking intake and output on this patient.
25. a. Mr. A has been abusing alcohol, which will affect hepatic function. He is 60 years old and therefore has some degree of vessel narrowing.

    b. Because of the history of alcohol abuse and the age of the patient, medication dosing may be reduced to lessen the chance of toxicity.

    c. The nurse should assess the renal system. If renal blood flow has been impaired, then excretion of medications will be slow and side or toxic effects may be seen in the postprocedure period.

Chapter 6

1. Pharmacodynamics
2. receptor
3. Potency, efficacy
4. frequency distribution
5. 50
6. lethal
7. therapeutic index
8. lower
9. Efficacy
10. Antagonists
11. b   12. a   13. b   14. a   15. a   16. b
17. a   18. a   19. a   20. c   21. d   22. b
23. c   24. c   25. d
26. a. Determine the age of the patient. Identify how often the analgesic is used for pain relief and how efficacious the medication has been. Identify if the dosage is standard and safe. Evaluate the therapeutic index for this drug.

    b. Chronic pain related to history of migraine headaches

    c. Has there been enough time for the medication to be absorbed and distributed? Does the patient need a more potent drug? Is the agonist/antagonist formulation of this drug not appropriate for this patient? Are drug-drug interactions occurring? Are drug-food interactions occurring?
27. a. What antibiotics are the patients taking? Are the doses standard, safe, and potent? Have the patients taken the drugs long enough to consider the slow results unreasonable? Is this an efficacy issue?

    b. The patient exhibits the following signs of wound healing: well-approximated wound edges, no drainage 48 hours after wound is closed, no inflammatory response past day 5 after the injury.

    c. Wound edges opening, drainage, inflammation, pain, fever

Chapter 7

1. growth
2. development
3. holistic
4. prenatal, embryonic, fetal
5. infancy
6. toddler
7. preschool
8. school-age
9. adolescence
10. polypharmacy
11. a   12. e   13. c   14. b   15. d   16. b
17. a   18. a   19. a   20. a   21. d   22. c
23. b   24. d   25. a   26. d   27. b   28. a
29. c   30. b   31. c   32. c   33. c   34. b
35. d
36. a. The skeleton and all major organs are developed by week 8. Because substance abuse is a teratogen, all or some of the major organs and/or the skeletal system could be affected.

    b. The woman may deliver a neonate that has multiple developmental anomalies.

c. Drugs and other chemicals ingested by the mother may cross the placental barrier and affect the developing fetus.

37. a. Middle-age adults are sometimes called the "sandwich generation" because they are caring for children, grandchildren and aging parents.

b. They must opt for lifestyle changes such as limiting lipid intake, maintaining optimum weight, and exercising to overall health.

c. Cardiovascular disease, hypertension, obesity, arthritis, cancer, and anxiety

38. a. Polypharmacy

b. The chances for drug interactions and adverse reactions dramatically increase.

c. Although the nurse should avoid preconceived ideas that all elderly patients are physically and cognitively impaired, a careful assessment of hearing, vision, and mental status is necessary.

Chapter 8

1. health history
2. chief complaint
3. physical assessment
4. observation
5. Nursing Process

6. f	7. e	8. d	9. c	10. g	11. h
12. b	13. a	14. c	15. d	16. b	17. a
18. b	19. a	20. d	21. b	22. a	23. a
24. b	25. c	26. a	27. a	28. b	29. b
30. c	31. a				

32. a. At this age adolescents want to be like their peers, as displayed in their dress and lifestyle.

b. Yes, related to noncompliance to treatment of a potentially life-threatening condition with potentially long-term adverse effects to major organs of the body.

c. Noncompliance to treatment R/T failure to follow treatment regime AEB blood glucose levels of over 400

33. a. The priority intervention is to establish the need for and use of an interpreter to communicate with the patient. This will enable the nurse to communicate a plan of care to the patient and to reduce the chances for legal implications.

b. Language, culture, lifestyle, education, low income, healthcare beliefs

34. a. The potential exists for withdrawal adverse effects from the substance abuse and the potential to require additional medication for pain relief. Also there is a potential for noncompliance to treatment R/T drug dependency.

b. Patient will follow established plan of care as an inpatient and outpatient. Patient will enroll in a substance abuse recovery program and be in compliance with goals of the program. The desired outcome will be for a complete recovery from the trauma and substance abuse.

Chapter 9

1. Nurse Practice, ACT, protect the public
2. beneficence, maleficence, autonomy, veracity, justice, fidelity
3. reasonable, prudent
4. assessment, planning, implementation, evaluation
5. documented, done
6. right patient, right medication, right dose, right route, right time
7. principles, conflict
8. preventable, patient
9. verified, author
10. legal, ethical, medication errors

11. b	12. e	13. a	14. g	15. f	16. d
17. c	18. d	19. a	20. d	21. b	22. a
23. d	24. d	25. a	26. d	27. a	28. a
29. b	30. d	31. d	32. b		

33. a. Assessment is the first step of the Nursing Process. Subjective data (complaining of a headache) and objective data (vital signs) are both used.

b. The ethical principle of beneficence would ensure that only good would be done and would be included in the nursing actions for this patient.

34. a. The short-term goal for this patient would be to understand that extra medication should not be taken without a doctor's order while in the hospital.

b. Have the patient verbalize understanding of the short-term goal.

35. a. Risk for injury related to excessive anticoagulation as evidenced by increased dosage of anticoagulant medication

b. Implementation would include monitoring the patient for signs and symptoms of increased clotting time and elevated prothrombin time.

Chapter 10

1. holistic
2. perceptions, preferred modes
3. values, beliefs, practices
4. access
5. impotence
6. contraceptives
7. Science, medicine
8. Psychology, sociology

9. c	10. e	11. f	12. g	13. b	14. a
15. d	16. c	17. d	18. d	19. b	20. c
21. a	22. b	23. d	24. d	25. a	26. b
27. a	28. b	29. b	30. d		

31. a. Assess Mrs. J's cultural background, level of income, lifestyle, religious beliefs, use of nonprescription drugs, and whether there are other

environmental factors (such as the husband's alcoholic parents living with her) that may contribute to her child's future alcohol abuse, or influence her well-being. This patient should also be assessed for the possibility of domestic violence.

b. Alcoholism has both social and biological components. Some persons are more sensitive to alcohol based on their genetic makeup. Alcoholism may develop in people who are exposed to socially accepted drinking. It may be influenced by culture, environment, poverty, and traumatic experiences.

c. Referrals for this patient may include a community group such as Al-Anon or her church. She also needs to enlist the support of her nonalcoholic family. She may need referrals for WIC or other financial assistance. (If the assessment for domestic violence is positive, make appropriate referrals.)

32. a. Side effects of the antihypertensives should be assessed—especially whether they are causing impotence. Also, the patient's knowledge of the use of the medications and how to take them should be evaluated.

b. He should be instructed in the correct dosage schedule and side effects that may occur. The patient needs to know that abruptly discontinuing antihypertensives has been known to cause strokes.

33. a. Other types of pain-relieving measures that may be acceptable to this patient include guided imagery, biofeedback, acupuncture, therapeutic massage, heat, cold, and TENS unit usage.

b. Find out the patient's religion and offer her the option of a consultation with a minister regarding the use of stronger medications. Find out what she has done in the past to relieve her pain, and do this, if possible.

c. Possibly a nonnarcotic pain reliever would give some relief. Acetaminophen, aspirin, and ibuprofen do not cause the drowsiness often associated with narcotics.

Chapter 11

1. healing power
2. reduce, medications
3. judgmental
4. woody tissue, stems, bark
5. active chemicals
6. dozens, identified
7. Dietary Supplement Health and Education (DSHEA)

8. e	9. b	10. a	11. c	12. d	13. e
14. d	15. d	16. a	17. b	18. b	19. b
20. d	21. e	22. c	23. d	24. c	25. a
26. c	27. d	28. d	29. c	30. b	31. c
32. b	33. a	34. d	35. a	36. a	37. d
38. a	39. b				

40. a. The nurse should find out what herbs the patient is planning on using, and determine whether he is aware of possible side effects and herb-drug interactions.

b. Many herbal supplements cause increased effects from warfarin and digoxin. The patient should be informed that he may experience increased tendency to bleed and possibly digitalis toxicity. Herbal preparations should not be taken without consulting his physician. Since the patient may take the herbals in spite of the nurse's warning he should be instructed in signs and symptoms to report. Symptoms of bleeding include bruises, bleeding gums, and hematuria. Digitoxicity symptoms include anorexia, nausea, and yellow haloes around objects.

c. Some patients may be allergic to one of the many chemicals in herbals. Patients should start by using the smallest amount possible until it is determined whether they have an allergy to any component of the substance.

41. a. The patient may be experiencing serotonin syndrome caused by the combination of the Prozac and the St. John's wort.

b. Combining St. John's wort with tricyclic antidepressants such as Elavil or Tofranil may cause serotonin syndrome. MAOIs in combination with St. John's wort may cause hypertensive crisis.

42. a. You would want to monitor liver function studies (AST, ALT) because the combination of echinacea and methotrexate may result in hepatotoxicity.

b. Because this patient is already combining a prescription drug with an herbal that is known to have an adverse interaction, the possibility of herb-drug interactions should be stressed. The patient should also be made aware that herbal supplements are not FDA tested and may not do what they claim to do. He should be made aware of the possibility of an allergic reaction to an ingredient in the preparation.

c. This goal is probably not realistic, as the patient is already using an herbal preparation, although he is not happy with the results at the present time. The nurse should attempt to understand what the patient is trying to accomplish by using the herbal preparation and be prepared to offer him alternatives to meet his needs. He may need a new prescription, or possibly wish to combine herbals with prescription medications. Open communication and a nonjudgmental attitude on the part of the nurse will encourage the patient to explore possibilities and decide upon what is best for his situation. A more realistic goal might be to have the patient verbalize possible herb-drug interactions related to the echinacea prior to discharge.

Chapter 12

1. alcohol, nicotine
2. opium, marijuana, cocaine
3. dose, length of therapy
4. physical dependence, psychological dependence
5. Substance dependence
6. crack cocaine

7. benzodiazepine

8. methadone

9. tolerance

10. I (one)

11. Nicotine

12. withdrawal

13. a 14. c 15. c 16. d 17. b 18. b

19. d 20. a 21. c 22. a 23. a 24. b

25. a 26. a 27. b 28. a 29. b 30. b

31. c 32. a 33. d 34. d 35. c 36. d

37. a 38. d 39. b

40. a. Marijuana can cause lung damage and the chance for cancer of the lung.

b. Marijuana causes psychological dependence. It is also considered the "gateway" drug: It opens the patient to opportunities for poor judgment and the possibility of taking other drugs when the person is "high" on marijuana.

c. Lung cancer is a risk in those people who smoke marijuana.

41. a. There is substantial evidence to suggest that genetics plays a major role in addiction. However, many factors could increase the likelihood of someone abusing alcohol, as well as other addictive drugs. If a person has a genetic predisposition to substance abuse, it is best to carefully weigh the risks of addiction before consuming alcohol or other addicting substances.

b. When did the patient last consume alcohol? How much alcohol is usually consumed in a day/week? Has the patient ever had withdrawal symptoms? Has the patient ever been to an alcohol treatment program? What is the patient's current mental status? What is the patient's nutritional status? What is skin integrity like?

c. One nursing diagnosis is chronic low self-esteem related to substance abuse. The patient outcome is stable self-esteem.

A second nursing diagnosis is compromised family coping related to substance abuse. The patient outcome is the family will understand the behaviors needed to support a drug-free family environment and cope with the recovery process.

A third nursing diagnosis is risk for violence related to altered perceptions and poor impulse control. The patient outcome is no violence experienced; altered perceptions are prevented or treated early.

A final nursing diagnosis is deficient knowledge related to lack of understanding of the use and abuse of alcohol. The patient outcome is the patient will express the causes and treatment of addictions and will be able to express the prevention behaviors necessary to be drug free.

Chapter 13

1. central, peripheral

2. autonomic

3. fight-or-flight, rest-and-digest

4. presynaptic, synapse cleft, postsynaptic

5. Norepinephrine, acetylcholine

6. adrenergics, cholinergic

7. parasympathetic, sympathetic

8. Adrenergic

9. adrenergic (or sympathetic)

10. Cholinergic

11. e 12. b 13. c 14. d 15. a 16. c

17. b 18. a 19. e 20. d 21. b 22. c

23. a 24. d 25. c 26. d 27. d 28. a

29. d 30. a 31. a 32. c 33. a 34. b

35. b 36. a 37. b 38. a 39. c 40. a

41. c 42. a 43. a 44. d 45. c

46. $\dfrac{20 \text{ mg}}{1} \times \dfrac{5 \text{ cc}}{10 \text{ mg}} = \dfrac{100}{10} = 10 \text{ cc}$

$\dfrac{10 \text{ cc}}{\text{dose}} \times 4 \text{ doses} = 40 \text{ cc/day}$

47. $\dfrac{0.3 \text{ mg}}{1} \times \dfrac{1 \text{ ml}}{0.6 \text{ mg}} = \dfrac{0.3}{0.6} = 0.50 \text{ ml}$

48.

Drug	Class	Effect or Action	Interactions	
Benadryl	Anticholinergic	Dries secretions causing difficulty for patients with COPD	Increases heart rate and blood pressure	Causes drowsiness Urinary hesitancy and retention
Propranolol	Adrenergic blocker	Decreases bronchodilation causing difficulty for COPD patients	Decreases heart rate and blood pressure Causes orthostatic hypotension	Causes drowsiness and possible depression
Prazocin	Adrenergic blocker	Decreases bronchodilation causing difficulty for COPD patients	Vasodilation to decrease BP, allows increased heart rate	Urinary hesitancy
Proventil	Adrenergic	Bronchodilation	Increases BP and HR	

These actions work against each other in the cardiovascular areas and respiratory areas.

a. Potential nursing diagnoses would include:

  1. Ineffective airway clearance due to drying of secretions caused by Benadryl and interference with bronchodilation when propranolol is given with albuterol

  2. Possible altered urinary elimination: retention or hesitancy related to use of prazosin and Benadryl

  3. Possible altered cardiac output: decrease related to use of prazosin, propranolol

b. Nursing interventions that can be done to decrease possible problems or interactions include:

  1. Identify interactions and review with physician when appropriate.

  2. Increase hydration to 3 L/day to decrease risk of drying of secretions causing altered airway clearance.

  3. Monitor for signs of orthostatic hypotension, and possible decreases or increases in BP or pulse.

  4. Monitor intake and output to be sure patient maintains urine output and experiences no urinary dysfunction due to adverse medication effects.

49. a. To identify a nursing diagnosis, the nurse would assess the following:

  Muscle strength

  Knowledge of the medication regime

  Compliance with medication regime

  Unusual activities of daily living

  Unusual medical conditions

  Previous medications and present medications

  Administration of medications

b. Nursing diagnoses would include the following:

  Risk for injury

  Impaired physical mobility

  Knowledge deficit

c. Nursing interventions would include the following:

  Impaired physical mobility: assess for muscle strength and neuro status

  Risk for injury: assist for need for assistant with mobility; monitor for proper use of mobility equipment: canes, walkers, and transfers; monitor for safety hazards in home; monitor for ability to chew and swallow

  Knowledge deficit: monitor for patient's knowledge before and after teaching about medications, and safety teaching

Chapter 14

1. generalized anxiety
2. limbic, reticular activating
3. Anxiolytics, hypnotics
4. GABA receptor-chloride
5. benzodiazepines
6. Barbiturates
7. Respiratory depression
8. IV, III
9. Seasonal affective disorder
10. sedative and sedative-hypnotic

11. b	12. a	13. c	14. e	15. d	16. d
17. a	18. b	19. a	20. c	21. b	22. b
23. a	24. a	25. d	26. c	27. d	28. c
29. a	30. d	31. b	32. b	33. b	34. c
35. b	36. b	37. b	38. d	39. d	40. a

41. $\dfrac{1.5\ \text{mg}}{\text{dose}}\ \dfrac{1\ \text{g}}{1000\ \text{mg}} \times \dfrac{1\ \text{ml}}{0.001\ \text{g}} = \dfrac{1.5}{1} = \dfrac{1.5\ \text{ml}}{\text{dose}}$

42. $\dfrac{1\ \text{mg}}{\text{dose}} \times \dfrac{1\ \text{ml}}{5\ \text{mg}} = \dfrac{1}{5} = \dfrac{0.2\ \text{ml}}{\text{dose}}$

43. a. Nursing assessments prior to giving Versed include:

  Allergies to benzodiazepines or chemically similar drugs

  Liver and renal function

  History of any chronic respiratory conditions

  History of depression, alcohol or drug abuse

  Medications taken routinely and when taken last, including herbals

b. Nursing interventions would include:

  Resuscitation equipment, and airway

  Romazicon as benzodiazepine blocker

  Ventilator

  Someone to take patient home after the procedure

  Monitor vital signs q5–15min especially respiratory rate and depth

  Monitor patient's level of consciousness and responsiveness

c. To evaluate the effectiveness of intervention, the nurse would use the following:

  The patient has no injury related to the administration of Versed.

  The patient has normal vital signs during the administration of Versed.

44. a. Sleep pattern disturbance related to anxiety response

b. Interventions include:

  Explore potential contributing factors

  Maintain bedtime routine as per patient preference

  Provide comfort measures to induce sleep:

    Nonpharmacologic techniques

    Back rub

    Light bedtime snack

    Establish a regular time to sleep

    Avoid napping during the day

Decrease caffeine, chocolate, nicotine, and other stimulants in the second half of the day

Limit alcohol consumption

Exercise at least 2–3 hours before bedtime

Hot bath 1 hour before sleep

Comfortable sleeping environment

Use stress reduction and relaxation just prior to sleep

Relief of pain or discomfort prior to sleep

c. Pharmacological techniques will provide information to patient regarding pharmacotherapeutics. Benzodiazepines would be the drug of first choice for sleep. However, all of these drugs will cause interruption of REM sleep and, therefore, should not be continued for more than 1 week. Certain over-the-counter drugs are normally anticholinergics and again interrupt REM sleep, can cause a hangover, and should not be used for more than 1 week.

Chapter 15

1. acute, chronic
2. infection, trauma, metabolic disorders, vascular diseases, neoplastic disorders
3. oral contraceptives
4. folate
5. sleep, strobe, flickering
6. Febrile, 3, 5 fever (or temperature)
7. Tegretol
8. Partial, complete
9. Zarontin
10. Valium (diazepam), Dilantin (phenytoin)
11. Status epilepticus, respirations (or breathing)
12. brain
13. airway
14. seizures
15. abnormal, suppress
16. 3, months

17. f	18. e	19. b	20. a	21. c	22. g
23. d	24. a	25. a	26. b	27. a	28. b
29. c	30. d	31. c	32. b	33. b	34. a
35. d	36. a	37. d	38. d	39. c	40. b
41. a	42. b	43. d	44. c	45. c	46. a
47. a					

48. $\dfrac{60 \text{ mg}}{\text{dose}} \times \dfrac{5 \text{ ml}}{20 \text{ mg}} = \dfrac{300}{20} = \dfrac{15 \text{ ml}}{\text{dose}}$

49. $\dfrac{1200 \text{ mg}}{4 \text{ doses}} = 300 \text{ mg/dose}$

50. a. Possible risk of injury related to medication administration: Inappropriate administration of Dilantin IV can lead to emboli, hypoventilation, hypotension, venous irritation, seizures, or decreased level of consiousness.

b. Nursing interventions for administration of Dilantin IV:

Use saline only to mix Dilantin.

Infuse no faster than 50 mg/min.

Use IV line with filter.

Check for infiltration often as it is a soft tissue irritant.

Use large vein or central venous catheter only.

Never use dilantin IM.

Avoid hand veins to prevent local vasoconstriction.

Prime IV line with saline if hanging piggyback.

Monitor for LOC changes after seizure.

Keep side rails up and padded.

Have emergency equipment available.

Monitor for hypotension or depressed respirations during administration.

51. a. Top priority diagnosis: knowledge deficit related to new medical condition and new medication for management of seizures as evidenced by patient asking questions

b. Interventions:

Assess what the patient knows about epilepsy, seizures, and management.

Assess for any misunderstandings about medication and treatment regime.

Provide information to patient regarding the following:

Medications will be dosed at the lowest dosage to prevent seizures which will decrease the amount of side effects expected.

The medication dosages will be increased as needed if seizures continue.

Other medications might be added or drugs might be changed as needed to control seizures.

Seizures will be controlled best if patients are compliant with the medication schedule.

Patients will need to return for lab appointments and follow-up physician visit to evaluate therapeutic effect.

Side effects that might be expected initially include dizziness, ataxia, diplopia, and a change of urine color to pink, red, or brown.

The dizziness and drowsiness will decrease as the medication is continued.

More serious side effects should be reported to the physician.

Drugs to avoid: Many meds interact with phenytoin. The patient must inform the physician that he is on phenytoin before any medications are added. The pharmacist might also be consulted before over-the-counter medications and herbals or supplements are added.

No foods need to be avoided, but supplements of folic acid, calcium, and vitamin D will impair the dilantin. The nurse should give the patient a list of foods that contain folic acid, calcium, and vitamin D. These foods should not be taken in large quantities, although they do not need to be avoided.

Chapter 16

1. affective
2. major depression, bipolar disorder
3. tricyclic antidepressant (TCA), selective serotonin reuptake inhibitor (SSRI), monoamine oxidase inhibitor (MAOI)
4. SSRIs
5. TCAs
6. lithium
7. attention-deficit disorder (ADHD)
8. CNS stimulants
9. Seasonal affective
10. mood stabilizers, mania, depression

11. f	12. e	13. d	14. b	15. c	16. a
17. a	18. c	19. b	20. e	21. d	22. d
23. c	24. e	25. b	26. a	27. d	28. c
29. d	30. d	31. d	32. d	33. d	34. c
35. c	36. b	37. d	38. b	39. a	40. c
41. b	42. d	43. c	44. a	45. b	46. a
47. d					

48. $\dfrac{1.2\text{ g}}{\text{day}} \times \dfrac{1000\text{ mg}}{1\text{ g}} \times \dfrac{1\text{ capsule}}{300\text{ mg}} = \dfrac{1,200}{300} = 4$ capsules

$\dfrac{4\text{ capsules}}{4\text{ doses}} = \dfrac{1\text{ capsule}}{\text{dose}}$

49. $\dfrac{45\text{ mg}}{\text{day}} \times \dfrac{5\text{ ml}}{20\text{ mg}} = \dfrac{225}{20} = \dfrac{11.25\text{ ml}}{\text{day}}$

50. a. Risk for injury related to adverse effects of lithium

b. The nurse should assess for the following:

Knowledge of side effects: dizziness, drowsiness, nausea, metallic taste, tremors, vomiting, and diarrhea

Lab studies: renal and kidney function, blood levels of lithium

Interactions: diuretics and low-sodium diet possibly leading to lithium toxicity

History: allergies or previous renal or cardiac conditions

Mental and emotional status: previous suicide attempts or present intent

Knowledge of who to notify in case of adverse or toxic effects of lithium

Knowledge of adverse and toxic effects of lithium

c. The goal is to demonstrate the following:

Understanding of drug effects and precautions

Improvement in mood stability

Ability to notify or seek help when questions or problems arise

No injury related to adverse effects of lithium

51.

Goals for the Patient Patient will show (or report):	*Evaluation*
Improved affect or mood	No longer has suicidal ideation
	Engages in normal daily activities
Improved sleep patterns	Can sleep through the night, stays asleep, and falls asleep easily
Decreasing episodes of side effects	Decreased headaches, nausea, drowsiness since beginning medications
Continuation of medication regimen	Continues to take medications as ordered

Chapter 17

1. schizophrenia
2. chronic, acute
3. months to years, hours to days
4. positive, negative
5. cause (etiology), brain damage, medication overdose, depression, alcoholism, genetics, drug addiction
6. hallucinations, delusions, disorganized thoughts, disorganized speech patterns
7. interest, motivation, responsiveness, pleasure
8. antipsychotic
9. dopamine (D2)
10. schizophrenia, extrapyramidal

11. b	12. a	13. a	14. a	15. c	16. a
17. c	18. d	19. b	20. c	21. f	22. b
23. d	24. g	25. a	26. e	27. c	28. h
29. i	30. b	31. c	32. d	33. b	34. d
35. b	36. b	37. c	38. b	39. a	40. c

41. a   42. c   43. d   44. d

45. $\dfrac{15 \text{ mg}}{\text{dose}} \times \dfrac{1 \text{ ml}}{25 \text{ mg}} = \dfrac{15}{25} = \dfrac{0.6 \text{ ml}}{\text{dose}}$

46. $\dfrac{200 \text{ mg}}{\text{day}} \times \dfrac{1 \text{ tablet}}{50 \text{ mg}} = \dfrac{200}{50} = \dfrac{4 \text{ tablets}}{\text{day}}$

$\dfrac{4 \text{ tablets}}{2 \text{ doses}} = \dfrac{2 \text{ tablets}}{\text{dose}}$

47. a. Interventions used for the diagnosis of knowledge deficit:

Assess patient's readiness to learn based on the emotional response of the patient.

Provide health teaching related to Clozaril:

Can cause drowsiness, dry mouth, hypotension.

Does not cause as many problems with EPS as Thorazine does.

Get up slowly to prevent dizziness and falls due to orthostatic hypotension.

Avoid activities requiring mental alertness until effects of medication are known.

Avoid alcohol and other CNS depressants.

Weekly labs are required to monitor for agranulocytosis.

Report any evidence of infection: sore throat and mild fever.

Instruct patient on best time to take the medication and what to do for missed doses.

b. Evaluation will include the following:

Patient will report to lab and physician appointments as requested for lab work.

Patient will not experience injury (falls) related to dizziness, sedation, ataxia.

Patient remains compliant with therapeutic regimen prescribed.

Patient verbalizes understanding of medical regimen, adverse effects of medication, and need to be compliant.

48. Assessments include the following:

Vital signs: temp, pulse, blood pressure, and body weight

Behavior and appearances: dietary intake, activities of daily living, and socialization with others

Symptoms of condition: hallucinations, delusions, enjoyment of life, personal hygiene, speech patterns, and motor movement

Monitoring for side effects and adverse effects of medications such as akathisia, abnormal movements, dizziness, drowsiness, constipation, photosensitivity, or orthostatic hypotension

Let patient know that side effects will decrease with time on the medication.

Any past history of seizures; medication can influence the seizure threshold.

Assess plans for pregnancy or if any contraceptives are being used.

Monitor for fluid volume deficit by monitoring I and O, and weight, daily. Teach patient to increase oral intake to maintain hydration.

Monitor for improvement in symptoms of condition. Worsening of the condition should be reported immediately.

Monitor compliance with medication regimen.

Assess present medications or herbs that may interact with the new medication.

Chapter 18

1. autonomic
2. acetylcholine
3. Alzheimer's
4. Alzheimer's disease, multiple strokes
5. acetylcholine
6. genetic
7. antipsychotic, extrapyramidal
8. hypotension, tachycardia; muscle twitching, mood changes
9. cognitive, behavioral, daily activities
10. acetylcholinesterase inhibitor, functioning

11. b	12. a	13. c	14. a	15. b	16. c
17. a	18. a	19. b	20. c	21. i	22. h
23. g	24. e	25. f	26. a	27. c	28. d
29. b	30. a	31. d	32. d	33. a	34. a
35. c	36. a	37. b	38. a	39. d	40. c
41. c	42. a	43. c	44. b	45. d	46. b
47. a					

48. $\dfrac{100 \text{ mg}}{\text{dose}} \times \dfrac{1 \text{ tablet}}{25 \text{ mg}} = \dfrac{100}{25} = \dfrac{4 \text{ tablets}}{\text{dose}}$

$\dfrac{4 \text{ tablets}}{\text{dose}} \times \dfrac{3 \text{ doses}}{1} = \dfrac{12 \text{ tablets}}{\text{day}}$

49. $\dfrac{7.5 \text{ mg}}{3 \text{ doses}} = \dfrac{2.5 \text{ mg}}{\text{dose}}$

50. a. The nursing diagnosis is risk for injury related to drug effects and unresolved symptoms of parkinsonism. This diagnosis relates to sedation as a side effect of anticholinergics and of interactions with other possible CNS depressants such as Zoloft. The tremors and involuntary movements also cause possible balance problems. Orthostatic hypotension is also a side effect that causes instability of balance.

b. The patient will have no injury related to the side effects of medications or the condition (Parkinson's disease).

51. a. The priority diagnosis at this point would be risk of injury related to possible adverse effects of drugs and interactions.

b. Interventions would include:

Assess for interactions between medications in the regimen.

Tricyclics and benzodiazepines can potentiate their CNS depression causing sedation and sleep deprivation.

Assess for side effects of the medications:

Sedation, vomiting, diarrhea, obstructed urine flow, insomnia, abnormal dreaming, aggression, syncope, depression, headache, irritability, fatigue, urinary incontinence, and restlessness

Provide instructions for proper administration:

Give at bedtime and once daily.

Maintain a regular medication schedule.

Provide assistance to the patient when memory is impaired.

Assess for contraindicated conditions or medications:

Hypotension, bradycardia, hyperthyroid, peptic ulcer disease

Teach safety precautions for side effects of medications: no hot showers, arise slowly, have something to hold on to during ambulation when needed.

Include family and patient in management of the patient's condition.

Collaborate with other departments as needed: PT, OT, home health care.

Assess for caregiver strain.

Monitor for improvement with the patient's short-term memory or behaviors while on medications.

Chapter 19

1. narcotics, nonnarcotics
2. anti-inflammatory, antipyretic
3. unripe seeds of the poppy plant
4. tension
5. aura
6. nociceptor
7. anxiety, depression, fatigue
8. character, nature
9. stop, prevent
10. triptans, ergot alkaloids, serotonin

11. intracranial vessels, orally, parenterally, nasally

12. d   13. c   14. a   15. b   16. e   17. d
18. a   19. e   20. c   21. a   22. e   23. e
24. f   25. d   26. a   27. c   28. b   29. e
30. a   31. c   32. c   33. d   34. b   35. a
36. c   37. d   38. a   39. d   40. a   41. b
42. c   43. c   44. b   45. d   46. b   47. c
48. a   49. c

50. $\dfrac{400 \text{ mg}}{\text{dose}} \times \dfrac{5 \text{ ml}}{100 \text{ mg}} = \dfrac{2000}{100} = \dfrac{20 \text{ ml}}{\text{dose}}$

51. $\dfrac{0.4 \text{ mg}}{\text{dose}} \times \dfrac{1 \text{ ml}}{0.02 \text{ mg}} = \dfrac{0.4}{0.02} = \dfrac{20 \text{ ml}}{\text{dose}}$

52. a. Interventions include:

Assess the psychosocial situation of the patient because anxiety, fatigue, and pain will increase the sensation of pain.

Analyze the cultural aspects of the patient's pain.

Assess the knowledge of the patient about addiction and use of narcotic analgesics.

Teach the patient nonpharmacologic aspects of pain control: relaxation, massage, thermal packs, biofeedback.

Discuss the source of pain and the therapeutic management for the patient's pain, including using narcotic pain reliever only after less potent medications are attempted first.

Teach the patient to assess levels of pain with objective methods to quantify pain in order to better evaluate management of pain.

Teach the patient to journal to identify triggers for the pain.

b. The outcomes are the patient will report less pain after interventions and more relief from pain management techniques, both pharmacologic and nonparmacologic.

53. a. Interventions include:

Assess the medication regimen used by the patient.

Educate the patient on possible nonpharmacologic approaches: relaxation, biofeedback, massage thermal therapy.

Educate the patient on triggers that can cause migraines. Help the patient identify triggers that might apply.

Teach the patient appropriate administration techniques of the medications: Take Percodan as aura begins and not wait until headache is severe.

Teach the patient to evaluate the level of pain and evaluate the improvement using pain scale of choice.

Encourage the patient to revisit the physician if no improvement has been made with present medications. Encourage the patient to request or ask if additional medications might be helpful.

b. Goals include the following:

Patient will identify triggers to migraines and eliminate the triggers.

Patient will gain comfort by using nonpharmacologic approaches to migraine discomfort.

Patient will identify a decrease in discomfort after medication is taken.

Empower the patient to seek medication or measures in addition to those previously named.

Chapter 20

1. surface (or regional)
2. infiltration (or field block)
3. consciousness
4. IV, inhaled
5. pain following surgery
6. sensations, consciousness
7. location , extent of desired anesthesias
8. sensation, motor activity
9. opiates, anxiolytics, barbiturates, neuromuscular blockers
10. balanced, lowered

11. e	12. a	13. b	14. c	15. e	16. b
17. b	18. e	19. e	20. d	21. c	22. e
23. e	24. a	25. d	26. e	27. b	28. e
29. c	30. h	31. g	32. f	33. d	34. d
35. a	36. b	37. c	38. d	39. c	40. b
41. c	42. a	43. a	44. d	45. b	46. b
47. d	48. a	49. b	50. b		

51. $\dfrac{\frac{1}{6}\text{ gr}}{\text{dose}} \times \dfrac{\frac{60\text{ mg}}{1}}{1\text{ gr}} \times \dfrac{1\text{ ml}}{15\text{ mg}} = \dfrac{\frac{60}{6}}{15} = \dfrac{10}{15} = \dfrac{0.67\text{ ml}}{\text{dose}}$

52. $\dfrac{100\text{ mg}}{\text{dose}} \times \dfrac{2\text{ cc}}{200\text{ mg}} = \dfrac{200}{200} = \dfrac{1\text{ ml}}{\text{dose}}$

53. a. Knowledge deficit related to upcoming surgery and unknown medication regime

b. Interventions include preoperative surgical preparation and teaching:

Preoperative medications are given to relieve anxiety and provide sedation.

Anticholinergics are given to dry secretions to prevent pneumonia and aspiration.

Pain medications are given to aid in pain control.

An IV medication is given to cause rapid unconsciousness.

After IV medications take effect, the patient is given an inhaled anesthesia.

Muscle relaxants are given to provide relaxation during which time the patient will breathe with use of a ventilator.

Postoperative medications will include analgesics for patient, and antiemetics if needed to prevent vomiting.

Assess the patient's understanding of the information given.

Ask for patient questions.

54. a. The nursing diagnosis is anxiety related to anticipated pain of invasive procedure as evidenced by inability to concentrate; appearance of nervousness, apprehension, and tension; restlessness; and hyperattentiveness.

b. Assessment data include rapid pressured speech, tremulousness, restlessness, scanning of room, and asking questions.

c. Interventions are as follows:

Assist patient to reduce level of anxiety by reassurance and staying with the patient.

Speak slowly and calmly when giving information.

Ask about any physical problems and past history as well as present medications.

Give clear, concise information when teaching about the medications to be used.

Discuss alternate methods of relaxation.

Help establish short-term goals and reinforce positive responses to questions and actions.

Initiate health teaching in short, concise statements and move at the patient's own rate.

Monitor vital signs and any evidence of shortness of breath or chest pain.

d. Goals for the patient may include the following:

The patient will demonstrate a decrease in anxiety as shown by slower speech patterns, decreased vital signs, and the ability to repeat instruction-and-answer questions in a focused method.

The patient will relate information offered during the teaching session relating to the upcoming procedure.

The patient will relate information that has been taught throughout the teaching session.

e. Vital signs are normal. The patient repeats instructions and answers questions appropriately.

Chapter 21

1. essential (or Primary)
2. increases
3. increasing peripheral resistance

4. relax, decreasing

5. angiotensin II, aldosterone

6. Reflex tachycardia

7. fight-or-flight

8. Baroreceptors

9. diastolic

10. Diuretics

11. f	12. c	13. a	14. b	15. c	16. b
17. c	18. g	19. d	20. a	21. b	22. d
23. c	24. a	25. c	26. d	27. a	28. a
29. b	30. b	31. c	32. a	33. b	34. a
35. d	36. a	37. c	38. c	39. d	40. a

41. $\dfrac{15\text{ mg}}{1} \times \dfrac{2\text{ ml}}{20\text{ mg}} = 1.5\text{ ml}$

42. $\dfrac{60\text{ mg}}{1} \times \dfrac{1\text{ tablet}}{120\text{ mg}} = \frac{1}{2}\text{ tablet}$

43. a. Assessment data include smoking, overweight, elevated lipids, and anxiety.

   b. Nursing diagnoses are as follows:

   1. Imbalanced nutrition: More than body requirements (Outcome: Patient demonstrates accurate knowledge of dietary regimen to lower dietary fats.)

   2. Deficient knowledge: Purpose, precautions, and side effects of antihypertensive drugs (Outcome: Patient will verbalize accurate understanding of the purpose, precautions, and side effects of drugs used to treat hypertension.)

   3. Health-seeking behaviors: Relaxation techniques to effectively reduce stress (Outcome: Patient reports subjective relief of stress after using relaxation techniques.)

   c. The nurse will consider adding a second antihypertensive drug class if the first drug has proven to be inadequate in treatment of HTN. It is common to prescribe two antihypertensives concurrently to manage resistant HTN.

44. a. Orthostatic hypotension may be causing the dizziness. Explaining to Ms. F that she should sit on the side of the bed a few minutes before standing might solve this problem.

   b. Cardiac rhythm abnormalities are one sign of possible hyperkalemia. When switched to a potassium-sparing diuretic such as spironolactone, Ms. F should not supplement her diet with excess potassium.

   c. It may not be necessary to change this patient's medications, since it seems to be keeping blood pressure within normal limits. Patient teaching may be all that is necessary to resolve Ms. F's complaints.

Chapter 22

1. refractory period

2. Frank-Starling

3. 60

4. pump

5. preload, afterload

6. right

7. increase, strength

8. forcefully, slowly

9. digoxin immune fab (Digibind)

10. increasing

11. c	12. e	13. d	14. a	15. f	16. f
17. c	18. a	19. c	20. e	21. b	22. d
23. a	24. c	25. d	26. b	27. a	28. b
29. c	30. a	31. d	32. b	33. a	34. c
35. b	36. c	37. c	38. a	39. d	40. d
41. a	42. c	43. b	44. d	45. a	

46. $\dfrac{5\text{ mcg}}{1\text{ kg}} \times \dfrac{1}{1\text{ min}} \times \dfrac{75\text{ kg}}{1} \times \dfrac{1\text{ mg}}{1000\text{ mcg}} \times \dfrac{40\text{ ml}}{100\text{ mg}} \times$

   $\dfrac{60\text{ min}}{1\text{ hr}} = \dfrac{900,000}{100,000} = \dfrac{9\text{ ml}}{\text{hr}}$

47. $\dfrac{40\text{ mg}}{1} \times \dfrac{2\text{ ml}}{20\text{ mg}} = \dfrac{80}{20} = 4\text{ ml}$

48. a. Inotropic drugs affect the strength of myocardial contraction chronotropic drugs affect the heart rate.

   b. Cardiac glycosides and the phosphodiesterase inhibitors are examples of drug classes that produce positive inotropic effects. Drugs that stimulate beta$_1$—adrenergic receptors and anticholinergics cause a positive chronotropic response.

   c. In heart failure, you want the heart to expel more blood per contraction, thus positive inotropic drugs are needed. Positive chronotropic drugs are useful in treating cardiac failure and cardiogenic shock.

49. a. Hydrochlorothiazide and lisinopril will lower blood pressure, thus reducing the workload on the heart. Atorvastatin will help reduce blood cholesterol levels, which are associated with hypertension and heart disease.

   b. Mr. L is showing a need to control his life and manage his disease. He is 60 years old and he is determined to manage his disease without prescriptions. However, Mr. L should be encouraged to take the drugs as prescribed. He needs to understand that heart failure is a progressive disorder and that he is in the early stages. He can limit the progression with knowledge and attention to symptoms. He should be advised to try alternative therapies in addition to his medications, not in place of them.

c. Mr. L should be advised to continue his walks and develop a complete exercise and dietary program, under the direction of his nurse.

50. a. Labored and rapid respiration, coarse breath sounds with wheezing, rapid weight gain, and rapid heart rate support a diagnosis of heart failure.

b. The digoxin is given IV for a fast uptake and action. The 0.5 mg dose with a repeat in 4 hours is considered a loading dose. It is common to give an adult 0.25 mg/day by mouth of digoxin to treat heart failure.

c. This patient needs the renal system evaluated frequently. The output is of extreme importance, as retention of fluid will increase the heart failure. This patient had a 10-pound weight gain in 3 days. The nurse should be asking about the hourly urinary output.

Chapter 23

1. sodium
2. supraventricular
3. sudden death
4. supraventricular
5. atria fibrillation
6. pacemaker
7. cardioversion (or defibrillation)
8. arterial embolism (or small blood clots)
9. heart block, severe bradycardia, AV block
10. a. SA node
    b. AV node
    c. Bundle of His
    d. Bundle branches
    e. Purkinje fibers
    f. P wave
    g. QRS complex
    h. T wave

11. a	12. c	13. b	14. d	15. d	16. a
17. c	18. a	19. a	20. e	21. a	22. a
23. b	24. c	25. b	26. d	27. b	28. c
29. a	30. d	31. d	32. c	33. b	34. a
35. b	36. b	37. d	38. d	39. c	40. b
41. c	42. a	43. c	44. d	45. c	46. b

47. $\dfrac{100 \text{ ml}}{125 \text{ mg}} \times \dfrac{20 \text{ mg}}{1 \text{ hr}} = \dfrac{2,000}{125} = \dfrac{16 \text{ ml}}{\text{hr}}$

48. $\dfrac{250 \text{ ml}}{900 \text{ mg}} \times \dfrac{0.5 \text{ mg}}{1 \text{ min}} \times \dfrac{60 \text{ min}}{1 \text{ hr}} =$

$\dfrac{7500}{900} = \dfrac{8.33 \text{ ml}}{\text{hr}}$ or $\dfrac{8 \text{ ml}}{\text{hr}}$

49. a. Because propranolol decreases heart rate and slows conduction through the AV node, the nurse should document heart rate and rhythm before giving propranolol. The nurse should also assess for the presence of heart block, bradycardia, AV block, and asthma. A blood pressure assessment is essential before the delivery of propranolol.

b. Quinidine is an antidysrhythmic drug. It will slow the conduction and prolong the refractory period. The patient should be placed in the supine position because hypotension can result following administration.

c. Quinidine can cause diarrhea. It can also cause dysrhythmias or worsen existing ones. The nurse must therefore assess cardiac rhythm frequently. The nurse must also assess for dehydration and fluid and electrolyte imbalance because of the loss of fluid from diarrhea. A common side effect of propranolol is hypotension and bradycardia. The nurse must be alert for the patient's complaints of dizziness and fatigue.

50. a. Assess cardiac rhythm. Do not give if patient is demonstrating heart block, severe hypotension, severe congestive failure, or cardiogenic shock. Make sure vital signs and ECG are documented before drug is given. Note shortness of breath, presence of cough, chest pain, and urinary output.

b. Teach patient about heart rate and need to notify nurse if rate goes below 60 bpm. Watch for orthostatic hypotension, confusion, and chest pain. Do not give with grapefruit juice as it may increase the level of Calan. Hawthorne, a herbal supplement, can cause hypotension if given with Calan.

c. Nursing diagnoses include:

Altered tissue perfusion related to cardiac conduction abnormality

Knowledge deficit related to medication regimen

Risk for injury related to medication adverse effects

Chapter 24

1. a. prothrombin activator
   b. thrombin
   c. fibrinogen
2. a. plasmin
   b. plasminogen activator
3. embolus
4. anticoagulants
5. thrombolytics
6. Antifibrinolytics
7. prothrombin time (PT), International normalized ratio (INR)

8. a	9. e	10. c	11. b	12. g	13. c
14. f	15. f	16. e	17. g	18. d	19. a
20. a	21. c	22. b	23. d	24. a	25. d
26. c	27. c	28. a	29. a	30. c	31. d
32. d	33. c	34. b	35. b	36. d	37. a
38. b	39. a	40. b	41. a	42. d	43. c

44. $\dfrac{2500\ U}{1\ hr} \times \dfrac{1000\ ml}{50,000\ U} - \dfrac{2,500,000}{50,000} = \dfrac{50\ ml}{hr}$

45. $\dfrac{20,000\ U}{500\ ml} \times \dfrac{30\ ml}{1\ hr} = \dfrac{1200\ U}{hr}$

$\dfrac{1200\ U}{1\ hr} \times \dfrac{24\ hr}{1\ day} = \dfrac{28,800\ U}{day}$

46. a. Ms. S should use caution when engaged in activities that can cause bleeding, such as shaving, brushing teeth, trimming nails, and using kitchen knives. A soft toothbrush and an electric razor are safe choices. Contact activities, because of their high risk for injury, should be avoided.

b. Ms. S should report unusual bruising or bleeding such as nose bleeds, bleeding gums, black or red stools, heavy menstrual periods, or spitting up blood.

c. Aspirin or other medications containing salicylates should never be taken. Acetaminophen could be used for headaches. Feverfew, garlic, ginger, and arnica also should be avoided.

47. a. Alcohol abuse is a major irritant for GI ulcer formation. The chronic use of alcohol might contribute to ulceration. The use of warfarin also prolongs bleeding time, thus the bright red blood during vomiting.

b. Nursing diagnoses are as follows:

Altered tissue perfusion related to blood loss (Outcome: The patient will experience a stable blood pressure and pulse. The patient will have no signs and symptoms of anoxia.)

Knowledge deficit related to alcohol consumption (Outcome: The patient will demonstrate understanding of the long-term effects of alcohol consumption.)

Knowledge deficit related to warfarin treatment (Outcome: The patient will demonstrate understanding of the drug's action by accurately describing drug side effects and precautions.)

c. Immediate IM administration of vitamin K could reverse the anticoagulation effects of warfarin. Administration of an antifibrinolytic, such as aminocaproic acid (Amicar), might reduce excessive bleeding from the ulcer site.

Chapter 25

1. angina pectoris
2. plaque
3. stable
4. organic nitrates
5. transdermal patch
6. coronary artery
7. anticoagulants
8. clot, bleeding
9. removal of an existing clot, prevention of additional thrombi
10. percutaneous transluminal coronary angioplasty (PTCA), coronary artery bypass graft (CABG)

11. c	12. a	13. b	14. b	15. c	16. a
17. c	18. a	19. a	20. c	21. b	22. a
23. d	24. b	25. c	26. c	27. a	28. d
29. a	30. d	31. d	32. b	33. b	34. a
35. c	36. c	37. c	38. c	39. c	40. d
41. b	42. d	43. b	44. b	45. a	46. c

47. $\dfrac{50\ mg}{250\ ml} \times \dfrac{1000\ mcg}{1\ mg} \times \dfrac{1\ ml}{60\ gtt} \times \dfrac{15\ gtt}{1\ min}$

$\dfrac{750,000}{15,000} = \dfrac{50\ mcg}{min}$

48. $\dfrac{100\ ml}{125\ mg} \times \dfrac{60\ gtt}{1\ ml} \times \dfrac{10\ mg}{1\ hr} \times \dfrac{1\ hr}{60\ min} =$

$\dfrac{60,000}{7500} = \dfrac{8\ gtt}{min}$

49. a. His advancing age has put him at risk for atherosclerosis. His heavy tobacco use has predisposed him to vascular disease. His weight has increased the stress on the cardiovascular system. His life may be considered stressful based on the size of his family. He may have led a sedentary life because of his career path as an accountant.

b. Symptoms include slurred speech and weakness on the left side.

c. Retavase will dissolve the cerebral thrombosis. Lasix will control blood pressure and decrease the chances of further clot movement. Heparin prevents further thrombi development.

d. Hydrochlorothiazide is a diuretic that will treat Mr. M's hypertension. It is a safer drug for home use as it does not lower potassium like Lasix. Warfarin is taken orally and will be used to anticoagulate. This drug is used to prevent further thrombi development and therefore prevent an embolus event. Warfarin is a good discharge anticoagulant because it can be given by mouth. Diltiazem is a calcium channel blocker that is an effective drug to be used at home to stabilize hypertension.

50. a. Nursing diagnoses are as follows:

Altered tissue perfusion related to vascular disease (Outcome: Patient will experience relief of chest pain.)

Pain (headache) related to adverse effects of medication (Outcome: Patient will experience relief of headaches.)

Decreased cardiac output related to loss of myocardial muscle function (Outcome: Patient has adequate cardiac output within 24 hours of treatment as evidenced by BP <160/90 mm Hg, respiration < 20/min.)

b. Patient presents with some worsening signs of heart failure. Respiration is elevated to 28/min. Lower extremities are edematous, chest pain is not relieved, and patient is gaining weight.

c. The following reasons may be suspected:

1. Possibly Mrs. R is not taking the medications correctly. Review the medication delivery systems used to treat her chest pain and determine if she is using the medications correctly.

2. Mrs. R's medical situation may be worsening. Her coronary arteries may be obstructed and cardiac failure is occurring based on coronary occlusion.

3. Mrs. R. may be resistant to the nitrates; therefore, new agents may be necessary to treat her chest pain or current agents may need to be increased in dosage.

4. The combination treatment (nitrate, beta-blocker, calcium channel blocker) may not be the best combination to treat this patient.

Chapter 26

1. vascular
2. sympathetic
3. alpha
4. alpha, beta
5. beta$_1$
6. basic life support
7. Whole blood
8. circulatory overload
9. periorbital edema, urticaria, wheezing, difficulty breathing
10. PT, PTT, bleeding time
11. a   12. b   13. c   14. a   15. b   16. c

17. a   18. b   19. b   20. c   21. d   22. a
23. c   24. b   25. d   26. c   27. a   28. b
29. d   30. d   31. b   32. d   33. a   34. c
35. b

36. 13.86 ml/hr: 369.6 mcg/min

$$\frac{92.4 \text{ kg}}{1 \text{ min}} \times \frac{4 \text{ mcg}}{1 \text{ kg}} \times \frac{1 \text{ mg}}{1000 \text{ mcg}} \times \frac{250 \text{ ml}}{400 \text{ mg}} \times \frac{60 \text{ min}}{1 \text{ hr}} =$$

$$\frac{5,544,000}{400,000} = 13.86 \text{ ml/h}r$$

$$\frac{400 \text{ mg}}{250 \text{ ml}} \times \frac{1000 \text{ mcg}}{1 \text{ mg}} \times \frac{1 \text{ hr}}{60 \text{ min}} \times \frac{13.86 \text{ ml}}{1 \text{ hr}} =$$

$$\frac{5,544,000}{15,000} = \frac{369.60 \text{ mcg}}{\text{min}}$$

37. $$\frac{99.4 \text{ kg}}{1 \text{ min}} \times \frac{5 \text{ mcg}}{1 \text{ kg}} \times \frac{1 \text{ mg}}{1000 \text{ mcg}} \times \frac{250 \text{ ml}}{500 \text{ mg}} \times \frac{60 \text{ min}}{1 \text{ hr}} =$$

$$\frac{7,455,000}{500,000} = \frac{14.91 \text{ ml}}{\text{hr}}$$

38. a. Assessment data include auto accident, wandering, confusion, weak pulse, dysrhythmia, changing blood pressure, pulse, and unresponsiveness.

b. Altered tissue perfusion related to changing pulse and blood pressure

c. Dextran is an IV colloid given to expand fluid volume. If blood pressure rises, the nurse can assume the drug is effective. Norepinephrine is a potent vasoconstrictor used to reverse the severe hypotension. If blood pressure rises, then the nurse can assume the drug is effective. Dobutamine will help the heart beat with more force so that vital organs can receive blood and nutrients. When pulse becomes strong and blood pressure rises, the nurse can assume that the drug is effective. Lidocaine was likely given to correct the dysrhythmia. When heart rate and rhythm return to preaccident levels, then the nurse can assume the medication was effective.

39. a. With a closed head injury, neurogenic shock must be considered. The fact that the patient is comatose and has slow respirations, low blood pressure, and pulse, and has unresponsive pupils, supports this diagnosis.

b. Vasoconstrictors such as norepinephrine will likely be needed to maintain the patient's blood pressure; an inotropic agent such as dopamine may be useful in strengthening the force of the myocardial contraction.

c. Blood pressure, pulse, and respirations return to normal. The patient regains consciousness. No CPR is necessary and no tissue hypoxia results to the brain or kidney.

Chapter 27

1. hyperlipidemia
2. plaque
3. triglycerides, phospholipids, steroids
4. cholesterol, triglycerides, phospholipids
5. statins
6. 5   7. b   8. d   9. c   10. a   11. c
12. b   13. b   14. d   15. d   16. d   17. b
18. b   19. a   20. d   21. c   22. b   23. c
24. a   25. c   26. c
27. Zocor: 2 tablets at bedtime which is usually 2100 hours

$$\frac{40 \text{ mg}}{1} \times \frac{1 \text{ tablet}}{40 \text{ mg}} = \frac{40}{40} = 1 \text{ tablet}$$

28. Lopid: 2 tablets, divide the dose, give one in the morning 30 minutes before breakfast, and 1 tablet 30 minutes before the evening meal

$$\frac{1.2 \text{ g}}{1} \times \frac{1000 \text{ mg}}{1 \text{ g}} \times \frac{1 \text{ tablet}}{600 \text{ mg}} = \frac{1,200}{600} = 2 \text{ tablets}$$

29. a. Data assessment includes obese; history of two heart attacks; history of hypertension, elevated LDL, elevated triglycerides.

   b. Therapy with a statin drug is highly indicated because the patient has a history of heart disease and hypertension with elevated lipid levels.

   c. Reduce dietary intake of lipids and explain exercise program.

30. a. Ascertain if the patient is taking the drugs as prescribed. If she is taking the drugs, then dietary habit changes are important to discuss, especially lipid-rich foods. Many patients believe that if they are taking lipid-lowering agents, they do not have to watch their dietary fat intake.

   b. Teach risk factor modification which includes diet restrictions related to fats, calorie assessment, exercise assessment, stress assessment, knowledge, and understanding of when to take statin drug. Remember it is best to take statin drugs in the evening as the body produces the most cholesterol during the night.

Chapter 28

1. fluid
2. 200 billion
3. erythropoiesis, erythropoietin
4. epoetin alfa (Epogen, Procrit)
5. different types, leukocytes
6. platelets
7. size, color

8. Ferritin, hemosiderin
9. Transferrin
10. recycled
11. c   12. a   13. b   14. a   15. b   16. a
17. c   18. d   19. c   20. c   21. b   22. d
23. a   24. c   25. a   26. b   27. d   28. b
29. a   30. d   31. c   32. a   33. c   34. a
35. b

36. $$\frac{57 \text{ kg}}{1 \text{ day}} \times \frac{5 \text{ mcg}}{1 \text{ kg}} = \frac{285}{1} = \frac{285 \text{ mcg}}{\text{day}}$$

37. No;

$$\frac{66 \text{ lb}}{1 \text{ day}} \times \frac{1 \text{ kg}}{2.2 \text{ lb}} \times \frac{20 \text{ mcg}}{1 \text{ kg}} = \frac{1320}{2.2} = \frac{600 \text{ mcg}}{\text{day}}$$

38. a. Renal failure causes a decrease in the production of the hormone erythropoietin. This leads to decreased production of RBCs and anemia.

   b. Hypertension is the most likely side effect to occur. It is related to the increased hematocrit and also to the renal failure. Others include CVA, MI, and thrombophlebitis, all related to the increased hematocrit. It would be important to ask the patient if he had any blurred vision, slurred speech, transient weakness, chest pain, or calf pain during your assessment.

   c. Topics to cover include the importance of keeping physicians' appointments so that blood pressure can be monitored, how to self-administer SC injections, used needle disposal, reportable BP changes, and how to take his own blood pressure at home. Signs and symptoms of thrombophlebitis should be discussed. The patient should also be taught to maintain adequate dietary intake of iron, folate, and B_{12} and to maintain his renal diet.

39. a. He should tell you that the cause of pernicious anemia is due to lack of the intrinsic factor, in this case probably caused by his chronic gastritis. Since oxygen is carried on the RBCs and he is anemic, the body cells are not getting adequate oxygen. This causes the tired, lethargic feeling.

   b. The patient should be told to inform other nurses that he uses vitamin B_{12}, particularly in view of its interaction with colchicine. The importance of monitoring potassium levels should be stressed. Instruction on self-administration may be needed. If the patient gives it parenterally, signs of anaphylaxis should be taught.

   c. An iron preparation would be used in cases of inadequate hemoglobin or inadequate RBCs. The problem in megaloblastic anemia is that the RBCs are not maturing properly. B_{12} will treat this problem.

40. a. Assessments include health history, allergies, history of bacterial or fungal infections, vital signs, and WBC with differential.

    b. The patient should be told that filgrastim may cause an elevation in liver enzymes. It may cause an allergic reaction. Due to the stimulation of bone marrow cells, it may produce bone pain.

    c. She needs to wash hands frequently; limit contact with crowds and people with colds; cook all foods; avoid fresh fruits, vegetables, and plants; limit exposure to children and animals; empty the bladder frequently; drink more; and cough and deep breathe several times daily.

Chapter 29

1. diffusion, ventilation
2. nebulizer
3. emphysema, chronic bronchitis
4. respiration
5. 12 to 18; emotion, fever, stress, pH
6. constriction
7. MDI
8. Status asthmaticus
9. terminate, frequency
10. dextromethorphan

11. e	12. b	13. a	14. b	15. e	16. e
17. d	18. c	19. e	20. e	21. d	22. b
23. c	24. a	25. d	26. c	27. b	28. d
29. a	30. b	31. c	32. b	33. d	34. a
35. b	36. c	37. a	38. d	39. a	40. c
41. a	42. a	43. d	44. c	45. b	46. d

47. $\dfrac{50 \text{ kg}}{1 \text{ hr}} \times \dfrac{0.25 \text{ mg}}{1 \text{ kg}} = \dfrac{12.50 \text{ mg}}{1 \text{ hr}} \times \dfrac{6 \text{ hr}}{1} = 75 \text{ mg}$

48. $\dfrac{4 \text{ mg}}{\text{dose}} \times \dfrac{5 \text{ cc}}{2 \text{ mg}} = \dfrac{20}{2} = \dfrac{10 \text{ cc}}{\text{dose}}$

49. a. Assessment: Green thick mucus. Increased incident of wheezing and shortness of breath and wheezing worsening over 2 weeks.

    b. Assess respiratory status, respiratory rate, vital signs, auscultation of breath sounds, pulmonary function studies; peak flow, ABGs, and O_2 saturations.

    Fluids: IV if necessary, PO if possible: 2–3 L per day

    Head of bed elevated

    O_2 as needed to maintain oxygen levels in satisfactory level

    Administer beta$_2$-agonist and monitor for improvement and side effects

    Patient teaching to include:

Preventive inhaler (beclomethasone)

Fluids: 3 L per day

Notify physician for any increased dyspnea, wheezing, fever, change in sputum color or consistency.

Encourage compliance with meds and discuss side effects and ways to decrease side effects.

> Avoid environmental antigens that trigger asthma responses such as pollen, animal dander, dust, smoke, cold air
>
> Eat regularly using smaller meals more frequently.
>
> Receive yearly vaccines to prevent respiratory infections.
>
> Decrease or eliminate intake of caffeine.
>
> Avoid smoking

    c. Beclomethasone is a glucocorticoid used to decrease inflammation and prevent asthma attacks. Theophylline is a xanthine bronchodilator used to provide bronchodilation.

    d. Ativan is a CNS depressant that is used as an antianxiety agent to decrease the dyspnea due to stress and anxiety. Metaproterenol is a beta$_2$-agonist that will bronchodilate and relieve the dyspnea.

50. a. Knowledge deficit related to medication change evidenced by patient asking questions.

    b. Assess patient knowledge of the medications that she has been taking and of her condition.

    Teach patient about side effects of medications, reason for administration, and when to take it.

    Write instructions for patient to take home.

    Answer specific questions by the patient:

    Reasons for administration:

    Antibiotics are for infection in ear and lung. Take antibiotics as ordered until prescription runs out.

    Proventil Inhaler:

    Take only every 4 hours as prescribed.

    Be sure patient knows appropriate manner to set up inhalation.

    Proventil decreases wheezing and can be used to increase respiratory effectiveness.

    Need only to use Proventil until symptoms improve.

    Tylenol:

    Take for fever or pain, no more than 1 g q4h as needed.

    Robitussin AC:

    Guaifenesin with codeine: Guaifenesin is an expectorant. Take with at least 3 L of fluid per day. Codeine is a narcotic cough suppressant. Codeine causes drowsiness and itching.

Robitussin is used to thin and remove secretions. Do not drive while taking codeine.

Sudafed:

A decongestant used to decrease stuffy nose and fluid in the ear. May cause insomnia. Take only as directed on package.

Benadryl:

Not suggested due to its drying effect on mucous membranes in the lung.

Notify physician or return to clinic if worsening or no improvement.

Chapter 30

1. antigens
2. immune response
3. humoral, antibodies
4. active
5. passive
6. Smallpox
7. cytokines
8. biologic response modifiers
9. superimposed infections
10. glucocorticoids, antimetabolites, antibodies, calcineurin inhibitors
11. c   12. a   13. d   14. e   15. f   16. b
17. c   18. c   19. b   20. c   21. a   22. c
23. a   24. c   25. a   26. c   27. a   28. d
29. c   30. c   31. b   32. a   33. d
34. 72 hours = 12,272.73 mg

$$\frac{180\ lb}{dose} \times \frac{1\ kg}{2.2\ lb} \times \frac{150\ mg}{1\ kg} = \frac{27,000}{2.2} = \frac{12,272.73}{dose}$$

2, 4, 6, 8 weeks = 8,181.82 mg

$$\frac{180\ lb}{dose} \times \frac{1\ kg}{2.2\ lb} \times \frac{100\ mg}{1\ kg} = \frac{18.00}{2.2} = \frac{8,181.82}{dose}$$

12 + 16 weeks = 4,090.91 mg

$$\frac{180\ lb}{dose} \times \frac{1kg}{2.2} \times \frac{50\ mg}{1\ kg} = \frac{9,000}{2.2} = \frac{4,090.91}{dose}$$

35. $$\frac{100\ lb}{dose} \times \frac{1kg}{2.2\ lb} \times \frac{0.15\ mg}{1\ kg} = \frac{15}{2.2} = \frac{6.82\ mg}{dose}$$

$$\frac{6.82\ mg}{dose} \times \frac{2\ dose}{1} = \frac{13.64\ mg}{24\ hours}$$

36. a. The immunostimulant therapy may cause a spontaneous abortion.

b. Complications or adverse reactions include encephalopathy, depression, bone marrow depression, nausea, and stomatitis.

c. Side effects include hematuria, petechiae, tarry stools, bruising, fever, sore throat, jaundice, dark-colored urine, clay colored stools, feelings of sadness, and nervousness.

37. a. Immunosuppressants are used to dampen the immune response to reduce the possibility of rejection. The patient will need to take the medication as long as the organ is viable.

b. This class of drugs was developed to suppress the normal cell-mediated immune response. In lay terms, the medication you are taking keeps your body from rejecting your new kidney.

c. Adverse reactions include superimposed infections, bone marrow depression, alopecia, arthralgia, respiratory distress, edema, nausea, vomiting, paraesthesia, fever, blood in urine, black stools, increased pigmentation, and feelings of sadness.

38. a. Vaccinations have eradicated smallpox and poliovirus. They have reduced diphtheria and measles to a fraction of their occurrence prior to vaccinations. They keep our children healthy and reduce the chance for life-threatening diseases.

b. A.J. may have a red area and a sore spot where the shot was given, but this is normal. Severe reactions are rare and usually occur at the time of the shot when help is readily available.

Chapter 31

1. to rid the body of antigens
2. mucous membranes
3. antihistamines, glucocorticoids, mast cell stabilizers
4. antihistamines
5. sympathomimetics
6. Mast
7. H_2 receptors
8. nonsteroidal anti-inflammatory drugs (NSAIDs)
9. Glucocorticoids
10. Cushing's
11. a   12. b   13. e   14. d   15. d   16. c
17. a   18. b   19. c   20. e   21. d   22. b
23. a   24. c   25. b   26. a   27. a   28. d
29. d   30. a   31. a   32. c   33. c   34. c
35. a   36. c   37. a   38. c   39. d   40. b
41. b   42. b   43. d   44. a   45. c

46. $\dfrac{30 \text{ qtt}}{\text{dose}} \times \dfrac{1 \text{ml}}{15 \text{ gtt}} = \dfrac{30}{15} = \dfrac{2 \text{ ml}}{\text{dose}}$

$\dfrac{2 \text{ ml}}{\text{dose}} \times \dfrac{6 \text{ doses}}{1} = \dfrac{12 \text{ ml}}{24 \text{ hr}}$

$\dfrac{30 \text{ qtt}}{\text{dose}} \times \dfrac{6 \text{ doses}}{1} = \dfrac{180 \text{ qtt}}{24 \text{ hr}}$

47. $\dfrac{500 \text{ mg}}{\text{dose}} \times \dfrac{1 \text{ tablet}}{250 \text{ mg}} = \dfrac{500}{250} = \dfrac{2 \text{ tablets}}{\text{dose}}$

$\dfrac{500 \text{ mg}}{\text{dose}} \times 4 \text{ dose} = \dfrac{2,000 \text{ mg}}{24 \text{ hr}}$

Not a recommended dose. 1000 mg is recommended in a 24-hour period.

48. a. Empirin 2 in a combination drug of aspirin and codeine 2 mg. Aspirin is an anti-inflammatory/pain reliever and codeine is an opioid used for moderate pain. Ketoprofen is also an anti-inflammatory/pain reliever, but with higher anti-inflammatory properties than aspirin.

    b. Glucocorticoids are contraindicated when an active infection is present.

    c. Aspirin is irritating to the stomach lining and with its anticoagulant effect may cause gastric bleeding. Codeine may cause constipation, nausea, and vomiting. Ketoprofen may also cause nausea and vomiting.

49. a. The drug classification is nonsteroidal anti-inflammatory drug (NSAID).

    b. They have no GI side effects and do not affect blood coagulation.

    c. The nurse should assess for congestive heart failure (CHF), fluid retention, hypertension, and renal disease liver dysfunction.

50. a. Children under the age of 19 years should not be given aspirin (ASA).

    b. Children under 1 year should be given infant drops related to variations in the strengths in the preparations listed as "children's liquid."

    c. Aspirin when given to children under the age of 19 may cause the potentially fatal condition Reye's syndrome.

Chapter 32

1. pathogenicity
2. antibiotics, anti-infectives
3. mutations
4. Nosocomial
5. broad spectrum
6. Superinfection
7. penicillinase (or beta-lactamase)
8. Cephalosporins

9. Macrolide
10. aminoglycosides
11. a   12. f   13. b   14. e   15. e   16. d
17. c   18. b   19. a   20. g   21. f   22. b
23. d   24. g   25. f   26. b   27. e   28. c
29. a   30. c   31. c   32. d   33. b   34. c
35. d   36. c   37. d   38. d   39. d   40. b
41. b   42. b   43. a   44. d   45. a   46. a
47. c   48. b   49. d

50. $\dfrac{500 \text{ mg}}{1} \times \dfrac{1 \text{ g}}{1000 \text{ mg}} = \dfrac{1 \text{ tablet}}{1 \text{ g}} = \dfrac{500}{1000} =$

$\dfrac{\frac{1}{2} \text{ tablet}}{\text{dose}} = \dfrac{\frac{2}{1} \text{ dose}}{1} = \dfrac{1 \text{ tablet}}{12 \text{ hr}}$

51. $\dfrac{500 \text{ mg}}{\text{dose}} \times \dfrac{1 \text{ tablet}}{250 \text{ mg}} = \dfrac{500}{250} = \dfrac{2 \text{ tablets}}{\text{dose}}$

$\dfrac{2 \text{ tablets}}{\text{dose}} \times \dfrac{4 \text{ dose}}{1} = \dfrac{8 \text{ tablets}}{24 \text{ hr}}$

52. a. The widespread use of antibiotics often leads to resistant strains of bacteria.

    b. The longer the antibiotic is used, the higher the percentage factor of resistant strains.

    c. She may develop acquired resistance.

    d. It will most likely become ineffective in treating her infection.

53. a. Broad-spectrum antibiotics are prescribed until the culture and sensitivity tests can be performed and the actual microbe can be identified.

    b. Culture and sensitivity tests are performed to identify the microbe.

    c. Specific drug therapy can be selected based on which antibiotic would be most effective.

54. a. Adverse effects are formation of crystals in the urine, hypersensitivity reactions, nausea and vomiting, aplastic anemia, hemolytic anemia, and agranulocytosis.

    b. The nurse must carefully monitor the patient's condition and provide patient education.

    c. Encourage 3000 ml fluid every 24 hours to reduce the possibility of the formation of crystals in the urine.

Chapter 33

1. Fungi
2. sporotrichosis, blastomycosis, histoplasmosis, coccidioidomycosis
3. candidiasis, aspergillosis, cryptococcosis, mucormycosis
4. mycoses

5. dermatophytic

6. lungs, brain, digestive organs

7. superficial, systemic

8. azoles, ergosterol

9. Amphotericin B

10. orally

11. a   12. b   13. a   14. a   15. b   16. a

17. c   18. a   19. d   20. b   21. e   22. f

23. d   24. d   25. d   26. c   27. a   28. a

29. d   30. b   31. a   32. c   33. a   34. b

35. c   36. a   37. b   38. a   39. a   40. d

41. $\dfrac{150 \text{ lb}}{1} \times \dfrac{1 \text{ kg}}{2.2 \text{ lb}} = \dfrac{150}{2.2} = 68.18 \text{ kg}$

$\dfrac{150 \text{ lb}}{\text{day}} \times \dfrac{1 \text{ kg}}{2.2 \text{ lb}} \times \dfrac{0.25 \text{ mg}}{1 \text{ kg}} = \dfrac{37.50}{2.2} = \dfrac{17.05 \text{ mg}}{\text{day}}$

42. 100 mg/50 mg × 1 = 2 tablets per dose

43. a. The patient should consult her obstetrician concerning the best choice for her drug regime. Antifungals with less adverse reactions are more commonly used for vaginal candidiasis such as terconazole (Terazol) and tioconazole (Vagistat).

b. The foremost importance is to treat the problem without harm to the fetus. Therefore, the drug of choice would be the antifungal with the least adverse reactions and the least potential for harm to the fetus.

44. a. The recommended drug regimen is chloroquine (Aralen) 600 mg initial dose and 300 mg weekly for acute attacks; primaquine only drug for a total cure 15 mg every day for 2 weeks.

b. With low doses of chloroquine, nausea and diarrhea may be expected. Higher doses may lead to CNS and cardiovascular toxicity.

45. a. The patient will receive metronidazole (Flagyl) 250 to 750 mg tid.

b. Adverse reactions include anorexia, nausea, diarrhea, dizziness, headache, dryness of the mouth, and metallic taste in the mouth.

c. Amebiasis involves the large intestine.

Chapter 34

1. capsid, ribonucleic acid (RNA), deoxyribonucleic acid (DNA)

2. intracellular parasites

3. latent

4. antiretroviral

5. high active antiretroviral therapy

6. neuroaminidase inhibitors

7. protease inhibitors

8. DNA, contaminated blood, body fluids

9. Acyclovir

10. HCV

11. c   12. d   13. b   14. e   15. a   16. b

17. d   18. a   19. a   20. c   21. c   22. a

23. a   24. b   25. c   26. a   27. b   28. a

29. c   30. d

31. $\dfrac{100 \text{ mg}}{\text{dose}} \times \dfrac{1 \text{ tablet}}{50 \text{ mg}} = \dfrac{100}{50} = \dfrac{2 \text{ tablets}}{\text{dose}}$

$\dfrac{2 \text{ tablets}}{\text{dose}} \times \dfrac{2 \text{ dose}}{\text{day}} = \dfrac{4 \text{ tablets}}{\text{day}}$

32. $\dfrac{9 \text{ mcg}}{\text{dose}} \times \dfrac{1 \text{ ml}}{20 \text{ mcg}} = \dfrac{9}{20} = \dfrac{0.45 \text{ ml}}{\text{dose}}$

Use tubercular syringe.

33. a. The combination drug regimen is called highly active antiretroviral therapy (HAART). The goal of HAART is to reduce the plasma level of HIV to its lowest possible level; and to allow the patient to live symptom-free longer. HAART also reduces the probability that a virus will become resistant to treatment.

b. Classes include nucleoside reverse transcriptase inhibitors (NRTIs), nonnucleoside reverse transcriptase inhibitors (NNRTIs), protease inhibitors, and reverse transcriptase inhibitors (RTIs).

c. NRTIs build their own DNA preventing the viral DNA chain from lengthening. NNRTIs bind directly to the viral enzyme reverse transcriptase and inhibit its function. RTIs inhibit viral replication because reverse transcriptase is not found in animal cells. Protease inhibitors block the viral enzyme protease which is responsible for the final assembly of the HIV virions.

34. a. The vaccination may prevent the patient from getting influenza or reduce the severity of the symptoms.

b. The vaccination lasts several months to 1 year.

c. Amantadine (Symmetrel) is the drug of choice.

35. a. Transmission occurs through exposure to contaminated blood and body fluids.

b. Symptoms include fever, chills, fatigue, anorexia, nausea, and vomiting.

c. Symptoms include prolonged fatigue, jaundice, liver cirrhosis, and ultimately liver failure.

d. The current recommendation is universal vaccination of all children.

36. a. Judicious use of drug therapy is still warranted during pregnancy.

b. Acyclovir (Zovirax) is the drug of choice.

c. Adverse effects are nephrotoxic and hepatotoxic.

Chapter 35

1. carcinogens
2. tumor suppressor genes
3. chemotherapy
4. surgery, radiation therapy, multiple drugs, special dosing schedules
5. alkylating agents
6. folic acid
7. intravenously
8. plant extracts
9. hormones, hormone
10. Biologic response

11. d	12. e	13. g	14. a	15. b	16. c
17. f	18. a	19. b	20. e	21. b	22. c
23. d	24. e	25. d	26. f	27. a	28. b
29. a	30. d	31. d	32. a	33. c	34. a
35. c	36. b	37. c	38. d	39. b	40. c
41. a	42. d	43. a	44. b	45. a	46. d
47. b					

48. $\dfrac{20\ \text{mg}}{\text{dose}} \times \dfrac{1\ \text{tablet}}{10\ \text{mg}} = \dfrac{20}{10} = \dfrac{2\ \text{tablets}}{\text{dose}}$

49. $\dfrac{25\ \text{mg}}{\text{dose}} \times \dfrac{2\ \text{ml}}{50\ \text{mg}} = \dfrac{50}{50} = \dfrac{1\ \text{ml}}{\text{dose}}$

$\dfrac{1\ \text{ml}}{\text{dose}} \times \dfrac{4\ \text{dose}}{1} = \dfrac{4\ \text{ml}}{\text{day}}$

50. a. Tumors should be treated at an early age with multiple drugs and using several methods such as chemotherapy, radiation, and surgery when possible. If Mr. U had not sought medical treatment early enough, the remaining cancer cells could decrease the chance of recovery.

b. Drugs from different antineoplastic classes can be given during a course of chemotherapy. Different classes might affect different stages of the cancer cell's life cycle, thereby increasing the percentage of cancer cell death.

c. Administer drugs on a specific schedule to give normal cells time to recover from the adverse effects of the drugs.

51. a. Medications include antiemetics, benzodiazepines, serotonin receptor antagonists, and corticosteroids.

b. The patient should avoid crowds, unsanitary conditions, and other potentially infectious situations. Proper hygiene is strongly recommended.

c. Anorexia can be reduced by providing the patient with her favorite foods. A well-balanced diet should be implemented, including consultation with a registered dietician.

52. a. Tamoxifen causes initial "tumor flare," an idiosyncratic increase in tumor size and bone, but this is an expected therapeutic event.

b. Tamoxifen is a selective estrogen receptor modulator (SERM).

c. The drug is effective against breast tumors that require estrogen for their growth.

d. No, this medication is a pregnancy category D and has been determined to have adverse effects on the fetus. It should be given only if the benefits to the mother outweigh the risks to the fetus.

Chapter 36

1. alimentary, accessory
2. transport, enzymes, digestion, absorption
3. villi, microvilli, food/medications
4. peristalsis, smooth muscle
5. cardiac sphincter, esophageal reflux
6. chief, parietal, intrinsic factor
7. acidic, 1.5 to 3.5
8. erosion, mucous, the duodenum, small intestines
9. peptic ulcer disease, glucocorticoids, aspirin, NSAIDs
10. peptic ulcer disease, *Helicobactor pylori*; drug therapy, NSAIDs

11. e	12. c	13. a	14. g	15. f	16. d
17. b	18. d	19. b	20. a	21. d	22. c
23. b	24. d	25. a	26. a	27. b	28. b
29. d	30. c	31. d	32. b		

33. a. $\dfrac{60\ \text{gtt}}{1\ \text{ml}} \times \dfrac{100\ \text{ml}}{30\ \text{min}} \times \dfrac{60\ \text{min}}{1\ \text{hr}} = \dfrac{360{,}000}{30} =$

$\dfrac{360{,}000}{30} = \dfrac{12{,}000\ \text{qtts}}{\text{hr}}$

b. $\dfrac{100\ \text{ml}}{30\ \text{min}} \times \dfrac{60\ \text{min}}{1\ \text{hr}} = \dfrac{6000}{30} = \dfrac{200\ \text{ml}}{\text{hr}}$

34. a. 1000, 1400, 1900, 2200 hours

b. $\dfrac{2\ \text{T}}{1} \times \dfrac{3\ \text{tsp}}{1\ \text{T}} = 6\ \text{tsp}$

$\dfrac{2\ \text{T}}{1} \times \dfrac{15\ \text{ml}}{1\ \text{T}} = 30\ \text{ml}$

$\dfrac{2\ \text{T}}{1} \times \dfrac{1\ \text{oz}}{2\ \text{T}} = \dfrac{2}{2} = 1\ \text{ounce}$

35. a. Nursing diagnoses include risk for injury and knowledge deficit.

b. Risk for injury would be the priority due to existing confusion. Knowledge deficit is related to OTC medication to prevent further confusion.

36. a. Short-term goals are patient will be free from injury and will exhibit less confusion.

   b. Liver function tests need to be monitored as cimetidine and ranitidine are hepatotoxic drugs.

37. a. Nursing diagnosis is knowledge deficit due to new medications.

   b. Do not take OTC meds before checking with nurse due to drug-drug interactions.

   c. Antacids should be given 2 hours before or 2 hours after other medications due to drug-drug interactions and the effect of antacids on the gastric pH.

Chapter 37

1. stress; sights, sounds, smells
2. anticholinergics, antihistamines
3. emetics, Ipecac, vomiting
4. Anorexiants, moderate
5. frequency, bowel movements
6. food intake, dietary fiber
7. impaction, obstruction
8. laxative, defecation
9. monitoring, education
10. esophageal obstruction, intestinal obstruction, fecal impaction; bowel
11. b   12. g   13. e   14. a   15. d   16. f
17. c   18. c   19. c   20. a   21. d   22. c
23. a   24. a   25. d   26. b   27. b   28. c
29. c   30. d   31. c   32. a

33. a. $\dfrac{10 \text{ mg}}{\text{dose}} \times \dfrac{2 \text{ ml}}{25 \text{ mg}} = \dfrac{20}{25} = \dfrac{0.8 \text{ ml}}{\text{dose}}$

   b. 3 ml syringe

   c. For average size adult, 20–21 gauge, 1–1 1/2" needle.

34. $\dfrac{2.5 \text{ mg}}{\text{dose}} \times \dfrac{4 \text{ dose}}{\text{day}} = \dfrac{10 \text{ mg}}{\text{day}}$

35. a. Risk for injury and knowledge deficit are two important nursing diagnoses for this patient.

   b. Patient will be free from physical injury related to frequency of stools and physical weakness. Patient will understand the signs and symptoms of complications and report them appropriately.

   c. Nursing actions include providing a clutter-free environment with commode at bedside and a call bell within reach, and monitoring for stools—amount and character.

   d. Criteria include abdominal assessment for presence of bowel sounds, palpation for softness of and pain-free abdomen, and act of defecation.

36. a. Initial assessment will include vital signs, evidence of weakness or confusion, and abdominal assessment.

   b. Objective data include vital signs, abdominal assessment, number of stools visualized with color, and character of stool.

   c. Safety issues are call bell within reach; ability to follow directions and call for help; commode at bedside, clutter-free environment with slippers available.

37. a. Initial assessment will include vital signs, adequate nutrition, absence of vomiting, stable laboratory studies, and lack of uterine contractions.

   b. The primary goal is a full-term pregnancy without harm to fetus or mother.

   c. Compazine is a pregnancy category C, so the risks must be weighed as fetal harm in animals has been noted.

   d. Outcome criteria will include: 1). VS and wt (no further loss of weight), 2). laboratory results (stable electrolytes), Hgb and Hct, 3). I&O (adequate nutrition and hydration).

38. a. Low-fat diet should be maintained while on Xenical and fat-soluble vitamin supplements should be added to diet.

   b. Supplemental multivitamins with D, E, K, and beta carotene should be taken daily: psyllium may be taken at bed time to decrease G.I. side effects.

   c. Psychological support and patient education reinforcing the difference between hunger and appetite accompanied by diversional therapy. Nutritional consult is needed to assess for healthy foods among what patient likes.

Chapter 38

1. essential amounts, homeostasis
2. D, synthesize
3. prothrombin, blood clotting
4. lipid soluble; A, D, E, and K
5. Fat-soluble, intestines, liver
6. Dietary Allowance (RDA), minimum, deficiency
7. Hypervitaminosis; A, C, D, E, B_6, niacin, and folic acid
8. Alcohol abuse, thiamine
9. ergocalciferol, dairy products
10. Vitamin E, free radicals, membranes
11. e   12. d   13. a   14. b   15. g   16. c
17. f   18. d   19. a   20. d   21. a   22. a
23. c   24. b   25. a   26. d   27. a   28. a
29. a   30. a   31. c   32. c

33. $\dfrac{200 \text{ mcg}}{\text{month}} \times \dfrac{\text{ml}}{100 \text{ mcg}} = \dfrac{200}{100} = \dfrac{2 \text{ ml}}{\text{month}}$

34. $\dfrac{250 \text{ ml}}{4 \text{ hr}} = \dfrac{62.50 \text{ ml}}{\text{hr}}$

35. a. Pulmocare is specialized for respiratory patients.

   b. Protein and albumin levels will need to be monitored as well as electrolytes, glucose, and kidney function tests.

   c. The four types of enteral feedings are oligomeric, polymeric, modular, and specialized.

   d. The overall goal for this patient is to have his nutritional status meet body requirements.

   e. Nursing interventions include monitoring daily weights, intake and output, and lab values to determine success of plan.

   f. Evaluative criteria will include 1. Respiratory assessment (esp.® middle lobe to note clearing or absence of adventitious sounds; 2. Daily weights with maintenance of body weight and adequate in-take and output.

36. a. Patient will receive hyperalimentation with high-caloric intake, supplemented by vitamins and trace minerals.

   b. Impaired swallowing post stroke is the reason for the TPN. A central line is necessary for TPN longer than 2 weeks to avoid phlebitis in peripheral veins secondary to the delivery of a hyperosmolar solution administered intravenously.

   c. The short-term goal is the patient will be free from hyper- and hypoglycemic reactions.

   d. The long-term goal is the patient will receive adequate nutrition allowing for change to enteral feedings.

   e. The nurse will monitor for the following:

   Hyper/hypoglycemic reactions and blood glucose

   Respiratory status, vital signs

   Insertion site for signs of infection

   Daily weight and I&O

   f. Patient will not experience difficulty breathing, will remain infection free, and will maintain moderate weight gain.

37. a. For long-term therapy, peripheral veins are not sufficient due to phlebitis. A NANDA diagnosis is Nutrition, more than body requires.

   b. This type of feeding will be necessary for 6 weeks or more; patient will be infection free and maintain stable lab results.

   c. The patient can go home with home care support in the community.

Chapter 39

1. Hormones
2. pituitary
3. electrolyte

4. IV
5. cardiovascular
6. anxiety
7. with
8. infection

9. c	10. d	11. e	12. a	13. b	14. c
15. b	16. a	17. d	18. d	19. c	20. b
21. a	22. a	23. b	24. d	25. c	26. d
27. d	28. a	29. a	30. b	31. c	32. b
33. a	34. d	35. c			

36. $\dfrac{10 \text{ U}}{\text{dose}} \times \dfrac{1 \text{ ml}}{2 \text{ OU}} = \dfrac{10}{20} = \dfrac{0.5 \text{ ml}}{\text{dose}}$

37. $\dfrac{200 \text{ mg}}{\text{dose}} \times \dfrac{204 \text{ tablet}}{50 \text{ mg}} = \dfrac{200}{50} = \dfrac{4 \text{ tablets}}{\text{dose}}$

38. a. Thyroid preparations increase metabolic activity. They may elevate body temperature, increase heart rate, and reduce the patient's weight. The effects of thyroid medications increase when a patient is also taking insulin.

   b. The nurse should take a thorough health history, communicate findings with the prescribing physician, and teach the patient to report adverse effects promptly.

39. a. PTU may cause vital sign changes. The patient should be taught how to monitor these and to report changes promptly. This may require the purchase of necessary equipment. Risk of infection increases with the use of PTU. The patient must understand the importance of avoiding crowds and individuals with known illnesses. This may lead to feelings of isolation.

   b. The nurse can assist by encouraging alternative methods of communication such as the telephone and computer when susceptibility is increased. Since drowsiness may occur with the use of this medication, teaching concerning safety is of importance. The nurse should instruct the patient to avoid being near environmental hazards, driving, and operating machinery.

Chapter 40

1. type 1 diabetes mellitus, type 2 diabetes mellitus
2. oral hypoglycemics
3. resistant
4. blood glucose
5. severe epigastric pain
6. Alcohol

7. b	8. c	9. a	10. c	11. b	12. a
13. a	14. c	15. c	16. d	17. d	18. d
19. b	20. a	21. b	22. c	23. c	24. b
25. a	26. b	27. a			

28. 35 U + 20 U = 55 U

29. $$\frac{10 \text{ mg}}{\text{dose}} \times \frac{1 \text{ tablet}}{5 \text{ mg}} = \frac{10}{5} = \frac{2 \text{ tablets}}{\text{dose}}$$

30. a. Pharmacotherapy for type 2 diabetes is usually oral hypoglycemic agents, and lifestyle changes such as proper diet and increased level of activity will be necessary.

    b. Because Mr. D is elderly, these approaches may be a problem as older patients are not as active as the general population, and they do not easily comply with instructions for a change of diet. Additionally, if Mr. D has other physical limitations because of his age or if he is not able to receive proper instruction because of these limitations (seeing or hearing, for example), these could be obstacles to diabetic therapy.

31. a. The nurse must communicate to this patient the importance of avoiding alcohol, cigarette smoking, and spicy, gas-forming foods. He should weigh himself daily; observe stools for color, frequency, and consistency changes; and eat a diet low in fat.

    b. This patient needs fresh foods, but with a fixed income may be unable to afford the foods that are best for him. The nurse may need to refer this patient to social services, which can connect him with agencies that may be able to provide meals and transportation.

Chapter 41

1. Follicle-stimulating hormone, luteinizing hormone
2. menopause
3. conjugated estrogens
4. amenorrhea
5. progestins
6. prolactin, oxytocin

7. d	8. c	9. b	10. a	11. b	12. c
13. a	14. e	15. d	16. d	17. d	18. d
19. b	20. b	21. a	22. c	23. a	24. c
25. c	26. c	27. c	28. d	29. b	30. a
31. b	32. c				

33. $$\frac{100 \text{ cc}}{2 \text{ hr}} \times \frac{15 \text{ gtt}}{1 \text{ cc}} \times \frac{1 \text{ hr}}{60 \text{ min}} = \frac{1500}{120} =$$

$$\frac{12.50 \text{ qtt}}{\text{min}} = \frac{13 \text{ qtt}}{\text{min}}$$

34. $$\frac{100 \text{ mg}}{\text{dose}} \times \frac{1 \text{ ml}}{400 \text{ mq}} = \frac{100}{400} = \frac{0.25 \text{ ml}}{\text{dose}}$$

35. a. Ms. M has a knowledge deficit related to the prescribed drug regimen. The desired outcome is for Ms. M to understand the drug regime and manage her regime appropriately.

    b. Estrogen replacement therapy may be prescribed short term to alleviate unpleasant symptoms occurring during and after menopause. Hot flashes, night sweats, vaginal dryness, susceptibility to infection, erratic menstrual cycle, and nervousness may be reduced. The short-term risks of estrogen replacement therapy are bloating, nausea, vaginal bleeding, breast tenderness, and other common menstrual symptoms. The long-term risks of estrogen replacement therapy are ovarian cancer, gall bladder disease, and breast cancer.

36. a. The nurse must use this medication with caution and continuously monitor maternal and fetus status. Adverse effects of oxytocin include fetal dysrhythmias, neonatal jaundice, and intracranial hemorrhage related to possible fetal trauma. Maternal effects include cardiac arrhythmias, hypertensive episodes, water intoxication, uterine rupture or uterine hypotonicity, seizures, postpartum hemorrhage, and coma.

    b. Changes in maternal and fetal vital signs must be reported immediately and the infusion stopped. Intake and output should be monitored closely. Contraction status during labor and fundal checks in the postpartum period are of utmost importance. The nurse must understand that uterine hypotonicity in the postpartum period is related to postpartum hemorrhage.

Chapter 42

1. Anabolic steroids
2. virulization
3. sildenafil (Viagra)
4. Benign prostatic hyperplasia (BPH)
5. Androgens
6. X
7. Alpha-adrenergic blockers

8. a	9. b	10. c	11. a	12. b	13. b
14. d	15. a	16. a	17. b	18. c	19. d
20. c	21. a	22. a	23. d	24. b	25. c
26. d	27. a	28. b			

29. $$\frac{150 \text{ mg}}{\text{dose}} \times \frac{1 \text{ tablet}}{100 \text{ mg}} = \frac{150}{100} = \frac{1.5 \text{ tablets}}{\text{dose}}$$

30. $$\frac{4 \text{ mg}}{\text{dose}} \times \frac{1 \text{ capsule}}{2 \text{ mg}} = \frac{4}{2} = \frac{2 \text{ capsules}}{\text{dose}}$$

31. a. The nurse should teach Mr. E that the goal of finasteride (Proscar) therapy is to reduce urinary symptoms related to an enlarged prostate. Urinary symptoms such as hesitancy, difficulty starting the stream, decreased diameter of the stream, nocturia, dribbling, and frequency should be diminished. The nurse should explain to Mr. E that is may be necessary to take Proscar for the remainder of his life to keep the symptoms under control.

    b. To evaluate effectiveness of therapy, the nurse should devise a method of follow-up to assess the resolution of urinary symptoms. Mr. E should also be encouraged to contact his nurse if symptoms worsen.

32. a. The nurse should obtain a list of herbs used by Mr. S. If he uses echinacea in conjunction with androgen therapy, his insulin requirements may decrease, necessitating a change in his insulin dosage.

    b. Mr. S should be instructed to carefully monitor his blood glucose during androgen therapy and be encouraged to report symptoms of hypoglycemia such as sweating, tremors, anxiety, tremors, or vertigo.

Chapter 43

1. distal
2. distal, reabsorbed, secreted
3. nephrons
4. a. efferent arteriole
   b. peritubular capillaries
   c. proximal tubule
   d. distal tubule
   e. collecting duct
   f. loop of Henle
   g. Bowman's capsule
   h. glomerulus
   i. afferent arteriole

5. a	6. b	7. c	8. b	9. e	10. b
11. c	12. d	13. a	14. d	15. b	16. b
17. b	18. a	19. d	20. c	21. d	22. a
23. b	24. c	25. b	26. d	27. a	28. c
29. a	30. d	31. c	32. d	33. b	34. c
35. d					

36. $\dfrac{1 \text{ mg}}{\text{dose}} \times \dfrac{1 \text{ tablet}}{0.5 \text{ mg}} = \dfrac{1.0}{0.5} = \dfrac{2 \text{ tablets}}{\text{dose}}$

37. $\dfrac{100 \text{ cc}}{2 \text{ hr}} \times \dfrac{10 \text{ gtt}}{1 \text{ cc}} = \dfrac{1 \text{ hr}}{60 \text{ min}} = \dfrac{1,000}{120} =$
    $\dfrac{8.33 \text{ gtt}}{\text{min}} = \dfrac{8 \text{ gtt}}{\text{min}}$

38. a. Nursing diagnoses may include risk for injury, fatigue, and knowledge deficit.

    b. The nurse needs to monitor blood pressure and ask the patient for recent blood pressure values. Inquire about the patient's medication regime. Review potassium levels if available. Obtain more information about presenting symptoms such as onset, alleviating and aggravating factors, and intensity. Inquire about other symptoms of hyperkalemia including irritability, anxiety, and abdominal cramping. Obtain a 24-hour nutrition history including beverages.

39. a. It is important for the nurse to communicate to Ms. F the health complications related to untreated hypertension. Assessment of Ms. F's lifestyle and stressors is also vital information needed to create an adequate plan of care.

    b. Lifestyle activities to reduce blood pressure should be communicated to Ms. F. Many factors may contribute to high blood pressure. These factors are often difficult to manage and most patients require assistance to make the changes necessary to improve their health. Ms. F should be advised of the health hazards related to smoking, lack of exercise, obesity, stress, and alcohol consumption. The nurse should choose teaching methods appropriate for Ms. F's busy lifestyle. Handouts and written material will reinforce teaching and allow Ms. F to refer to the information at a later date. Follow-up appoint- ments can be used to document progress in making lifestyle changes. Support groups may provide Ms. F with encouragement and accountability.

Chapter 44

1. Crytalloids
2. 7.35
3. 7.35 to 7.45
4. alkaline content
5. Hypertonic
6. Hypotonic
7. Isotonic

8. a	9. b	10. b	11. a	12. b	13. d
14. b	15. b	16. a	17. d	18. b	19. a
20. d	21. c	22. a	23. c	24. a	25. c
26. a	27. c	28. d	29. a	30. b	

31. $\dfrac{1000 \text{ cc}}{8 \text{ hr}} = \dfrac{125 \text{ cc}}{\text{hr}}$

32. $\dfrac{8 \text{ g}}{\text{day}} \times \dfrac{1000 \text{ mg}}{1 \text{g}} \times \dfrac{1 \text{ tablet}}{500 \text{ mg}} = \dfrac{8000}{500} = \dfrac{16 \text{ tablets}}{\text{day}}$

$\dfrac{16 \text{ tablets}}{4 \text{ doses}} = \dfrac{4 \text{ tablets}}{\text{dose}}$

33. a. Aspirin and potassium may irritate the stomach mucosa. Also an extremely low carbohydrate diet causes the body to burn fats for energy, creating ketoacids. CNS depression may be caused by an impending acidosis. Ms. S has a knowledge deficit of her drug regime requiring nursing intervention.

    b. Ms. S could benefit from a thorough nutritional assessment and resulting weight loss plan taking her drug regime into consideration. Referral to a nutritionist may be necessary. The nurse should also ensure that Ms. S understands proper administration of her drug regime.

34. a. Symptoms of hyponatremia include nausea, vomiting, muscle cramps, tachycardia, dry mucous membranes, and headache. The nurse should obtain a baseline set of vital signs and monitor values closely. The patient should be asked about the onset and progression of symptoms. A diet history including beverages should be obtained.

b. A hazard of working outdoors is sodium loss through profuse sweating. Fluid replacement is critical to avoid hyponatremia. Mr. W should be encouraged by the nurse to consume adequate amounts of water or electrolyte solutions such as sports drinks. The early symptoms of hypona- tremia should serve as a signal to take refuge from the heat and concentrate on fluid replacement.

Chapter 45

1. movement
2. nervous, muscular, endocrine, skeletal
3. muscle spasms
4. analgesics, anti-inflammatory agents, antispasmodic
5. spasticity
6. dystonia
7. tetany
8. a   9. b   10. b   11. a   12. a   13. b
14. a   15. a   16. b   17. a   18. b   19. d
20. b   21. c   22. a   23. a   24. b   25. a
26. c   27. b   28. a   29. d   30. b   31. b
32. b

33. $$\frac{75mg}{dose} \times \frac{1\ tablet}{25\ mg} = \frac{75}{25} = \frac{3\ tablets}{dose}$$

$$\frac{75mg}{dose} \times \frac{2\ doses}{day} = \frac{150\ mg}{day}$$

34. $$\frac{20\ mg}{dose} \times \frac{1\ tablet}{10\ mg} = \frac{20}{10} = \frac{2\ tablets}{dose}$$

Yes–safe dose.

35. a. Limiting use of the affected muscle, heat or cold packs, hydrotherapy, ultrasound, exercises, massage, and manipulation may help to decrease Ms. H's low back pain.

b. Ms. H needs to know that dizziness, dry mouth, rash, and a fast pulse rate with palpitations may be noted while using this drug. Another but rare reaction is swelling of the tongue. She should not take this drug with alcohol, phenothiazines, or MAO inhibitors due to unfavorable reactions.

c. Ask the patient to rate her pain on a scale of 1 to 10 and see if improvement is noted after using the drug. Monitor muscle tone, ROM, and improved ability to do ADLs. These should increase if the drug is effective.

d. The patient should be instructed in proper body mechanics while lifting, sitting, or engaged in other musculoskeletal movement activities.

36. a. Ms. B needs to know that Botox injections are indicated for moderate to severe frown lines. They are not for crow's feet. She also needs to know that they will, however, smooth the lines between the brows temporarily, and must be repeated every 3 to 4 months. Although botulinum toxin is a poison in higher quantities, it is safe for use in tiny injections.

b. Side effects of Botox include headache, nausea, flulike symptoms, temporary blepharoptosis, mild pain, erythema at the site of injection, and muscle weakness.

37. a. Mr. P should have a thorough assessment of his physical condition, especially vital signs, skin condition, mobility or lack of it, neurological function, self-care ability, and nutritional status. The nurse should also determine the adherence to his medication regimen, side effects, and what outcome the family expects.

b. Physical therapy exercises might decrease the severity of his symptoms. These include stretching to help prevent contractures, muscle group strengthening exercises, and repetitive motion exercises. Surgery for tendon release or to sever the nerve–muscle pathway might be used in an extreme situation.

c. Mr. P and his family should be instructed to report any significant changes in his level of consciousness such as confusion, hallucinations, lethargy, and decreased speech ability. Also palpitations, chest pain, dyspnea, visual disturbances, and unusual fatigue should be reported to the doctor. Treatment should not be discontinued abruptly. Taking the medications with food should decrease GI upset. Decreased urinary output, distended abdomen, and discomfort should be reported. Dry mouth may be treated with sips of water, sugarless candy, or gum if patient is able to use this.

d. Family/patient need to be instructed on gentle ROM and other physical therapy as indicated by the physician. Safety measures include rearranging the home to decrease the risk of falls or accidents, and placing needed objects within Mr. P's reach.

Chapter 46

1. calcium
2. parathyroid, thyroid
3. vitamin D
4. rickets
5. osteoporosis, Paget's disease
6. parathyroid hormone, calcitonin
7. calcifediol, calcitriol
8. complexed, elemental
9. Selective estrogen receptor modulators (SERMs)
10. bisphosphonates
11. bisphosphonates, calcitonin
12. Disease-modifying drugs
13. uric acid inhibitors
14. b   15. a   16. e   17. c   18. d   19. e

20. c	21. c	22. a	23. b	24. d	25. e
26. c	27. b	28. d	29. d	30. a	31. c
32. b	33. b	34. d	35. b	36. c	37. a
38. d	39. c	40. a	41. d	42. c	43. b
44. a					

45. $$\frac{4 \text{ mg}}{\text{maximum dose}} \times \frac{1 \text{ tablet}}{0.5 \text{ mg}} = \frac{4}{0.5} = \frac{8 \text{ tablets}}{\text{maximum dose}}$$

46. $$\frac{400 \text{ mg}}{\text{dose}} \times \frac{1 \text{ tablet}}{200 \text{ mg}} = \frac{400}{200} = \frac{2 \text{ tablets}}{\text{dose}}$$

47. a. The symptoms the patient is experiencing are normal for his condition. Allopurinol (Lopurin) is used for gout flare-up and primary and secondary hyperuricemia.

b. To allay the pain, NSAIDs would probably be administered with antigout therapy. Medications could be administered with meals to minimize gastric upset. Other expected effects would include diarrhea and rash. Precautions would be taken to minimize these symptoms. Over a longer time, difficulty in urination may occur.

c. During drug therapy, laboratory tests (BUN and creatinine) would be ordered to monitor whether the kidneys are functioning properly. Fluid intake and output would be monitored. Since allopurinol may cause bone marrow depression, blood cell counts would be taken regularly. Liver function tests would also be ordered.

48. a. Patients with kidney disease are unable to synthesize the active form of vitamin D from the precursors formed by the body or taken in the diet. Calcium is not absorbed well from the GI tract unless there is adequate vitamin D so the patient may become hypocalcemic.

b. The patient should be informed that periodic liver function tests will be necessary, as well as calcium, magnesium, and phosphate levels. The drug should be taken exactly as directed so that toxic levels do not develop. Fatigue, weakness, nausea, and vomiting should be reported. Alcohol and other liver-toxic drugs should be avoided. Exposure to 20 minutes of sunlight daily will help increase the amount of vitamin D available to the patient.

c. Again, the importance of routine lab studies for calcium levels must be stressed. Oral calcium supplements should be taken with meals or within an hour after meals. The patient should be advised to consume calcium-rich foods such as dark green, leafy vegetables and dairy products.

49. a. Osteoporosis occurs when the rate of bone replacement is less than the rate of bone breakdown. People at risk for osteoporosis include postmenopausal women, those who use excess alcohol or caffeine, those with anorexia nervosa, smokers, inactive persons, those who lack adequate vitamin D or calcium in their diets, and persons using corticosteroids, antiseizure medications, and immunosuppressive drugs. The disease can be detected through the use of bone density tests.

b. Medications used to treat osteoporosis include calcium and vitamin D therapy, estrogen replacement therapy, estrogen receptor modulators, bisphosphonates, and calcitonin.

c. The patient will need to be instructed that alendronate (Fosamax) decreases the breakdown of her bones. The usual side effects are GI problems such as nausea, vomiting, abdominal pain, and esophageal irritation. The drug should be taken on an empty stomach once a week. To prevent the esophagus from becoming irritated, the patient should not lie down for 30 minutes after taking the medication. Patient teaching for raloxifene (Evista) should include the need for periodic bone density scans. Sudden chest pain, dyspnea, pain in calves, and swelling in the legs should be reported promptly. The patient should not take estrogen replacement therapy while using this drug. In addition, safety measures regarding falls should be discussed, as well as the need for weight-bearing activity and adequate dietary consumption of calcium and vitamin D.

Chapter 47

1. keratolytic
2. scabies
3. retinoids
4. emollients
5. pruritus
6. antibiotics, oral contraceptives
7. eczema
8. papules

9. c	10. d	11. e	12. c	13. a	14. b
15. c	16. d	17. c	18. e	19. a	20. b
21. c	22. b	23. a	24. d	25. d	26. d
27. c	28. b	29. b	30. d	31. a	32. a
33. b	34. b	35. c	36. d	37. c	

38. a. Lindane should be used cautiously in children under 10 years of age, and only if other pediculicides fail. Since this is the case here, the mother needs to know that lindane might cause local skin irritation and adverse CNS effects such as restlessness, dizziness, tremors, or convulsions. This usually occurs after misuse or ingestion. This shampoo must be kept out of the reach of smaller children in the household. It should not be applied to open skin lesions or used if the child has seizures. Mother should wear gloves while applying the shampoo, particularly if she is pregnant. The shampoo should remain on the hair for at least 5 minutes. Use of tepid water will decrease itching.

b. The child's school nurse or teacher should be notified, and, the parents of the child with whom she spent the night, and any other children who attended the sleepover. Anyone else with whom the child has had close contact (grandparents, for example) should be notified as well.

c. Children in school should not swap clothing or towels. Coat and hat racks at school may need to be eliminated to prevent the spread from one child to another. Combs or other hygiene supplies should not be shared, and bodily contact with an infected person should be avoided. Also, the child should not sleep with brothers or sisters until the problem is resolved. The nurse should stress that this is not a problem of social class, but simply an event that occurs when there is close contact.

39. a. You would ask the patient if he has had nausea, vomiting, chills, and headache, as well as assessing the amount of pain and extent of the erythema. Also ask about sunburn and tanning history, the amount of time the patient usually spends in the sun before beginning to burn, and if he uses sunscreen products. An allergy history is also necessary.

b. Soothing lotions, rest, prevention of dehydration, and topical anesthetic agents may help. The topical anesthetics may be chilled prior to application to increase the cooling effect. In severe cases, aspirin or ibuprofen may be used.

c. Medication should not be applied to broken skin. If this occurs, call the doctor. Prevent sunburn by decreasing exposure to sunlight, or by increasing the SPF number of the sunscreen. Wear a broad-brimmed hat, UV protection for the eyes, and a long-sleeved shirt if extended exposure to sunlight is expected during peak hours of the day. Sunburn results from overexposure to UV light and is associated with light skin complexions. Chronic sun exposure can lead to eye injury, cataracts, and skin cancer.

40. a. Causes of acne are unknown, although some factors associated with it have been identified. Overproduction of sebum by oil glands, keratin that blocks oil glands, and certain bacteria grow within oil gland openings and change the sebum to an irritating substance. This results in small, inflamed bumps on the skin. Other factors include male hormone, which regulates the activity of the sebaceous glands.

b. A mental health history should be taken to determine whether the patient has had a history of depression or suicidal tendencies. Patients with seizures who use carbamazepine should be identified as there is an increased risk for seizures. Also oral antidiabetic agents may not be as effective, so the nurse should assess for diabetes, heart disease, and elevated lipid levels. Prior to using the drug a patch test must be done to test for sensitivity.

c. He should be told to monitor foods and avoid those that seem to make his acne worse. He can be taught to keep a food log to help determine which ones these are. Products that will irritate the skin, such as cologne, perfumes, and other alcohol-based products, should be avoided. If severe inflammation occurs during therapy, the physician should be notified. Use of OTC agents should be avoided unless approved by the physician.

Chapter 48

1. blockage, outflow
2. open-angle glaucoma
3. miotics
4. mydriatics
5. cycloplegics
6. external otitis
7. otitis media
8. mastoiditis
9. cerumen

10. a	11. b	12. b	13. b	14. a	15. a
16. a	17. g	18. h	19. c	20. b	21. d
22. e	23. f	24. b	25. b	26. b	27. a
28. c	29. d	30. d	31. c	32. a	33. b
34. a	35. c	36. a	37. a	38. d	39. b
40. b	41. a	42. a	43. a		

44. $\dfrac{250 \text{ mg}}{24 \text{ hr dose}} \times \dfrac{3 \text{ doses}}{1} = \dfrac{750 \text{ mg}}{24 \text{ hr}}$

45. No need to verify the order—this is the standard way to administer pilocarpine in an emergency situation. (Of course, if you are unsure of anything, it is always best to check it out before you go ahead!)

46. a. There is no permanent cure for glaucoma. Medications will have to be used indefinitely. Several classes of eye medications may be used alone or in combination to control the intraocular pressure problem characteristic of glaucoma.

b. Xalatan is used to decrease the IOP. Side effects may include conjunctival edema, tearing, dryness, burning, pain, itching, photophobia, or visual disturbances. The eyelashes on the treated eye may grow, thicken, and darken. The iris may have color changes, as well as the skin around the eye. Generalized flulike symptoms may occur. The patient should remove contacts prior to administering and leave them out for 15 minutes. Wait 5 minutes between different eye medications.

c. Patient should be instructed to report any visual changes, and any changes in medications or new health-related problems. He should be taught the proper way to administer eye drops, and told to schedule them around his daily routines. Signs of side effects should be reported. He will need to know that measurements of intraocular pressure will be done periodically. For his safety, environmental lighting needs to be adjusted when dark, and may need to be dimmed if there is photophobia.

d. Intraocular pressure should be measured using tonometry at regular intervals to determine the effectiveness of the medication.

47. a. Additional assessments needed include Timmy's allergy history and whether his mother knows how to administer the drugs properly and is aware of potential side effects.

b. Mrs. B needs teaching regarding the correct use of ear drops and the fact that aspirin is contraindicated in young children due to the risk of Reye's syndrome. Teaching should include the following: ear drops are contraindicated in cases where the eardrum has perforated. This is the most likely cause of the drainage in Timmy's ear, and may be seen on examination of the tympanic membrane. Explain that

the bacteria present in the outer ear may be carried into the middle ear when the drops run in, thus increasing the chances of a further infection. Timmy's mother needs to be made aware that ear drops should be warmed by holding under warm water prior to administration. Also the child should lie on the side opposite the affected ear for 5 minutes after the drops are put in. If the child is older than 3 years, the pinna should be pulled up and back; if less than 3 years, pull it down and back.

48. a. Mrs. I probably has impacted cerumen (earwax). This would explain the mild hearing loss and a sensation of fullness with intermittent ringing of the ears. Other assessments to make would include whether she has a history of ruptured tympanic membranes, auditory canal surgery, or myringotomy tubes, as these would contraindicate an ear irrigation and the use of earwax softeners.

b. Initial nursing interventions would include removal by using mineral oil or an earwax softener preparation, followed by irrigation with a bulb syringe.